OXFORD MEDICAL PUBLICATIONS

Head Injury
THE FACTS

A guide for families and care-givers

ALSO PUBLISHED BY OXFORD
UNIVERSITY PRESS

Ageing: the facts
Nicholas Coni, William Davison, and
Stephen Webster

Alcoholism: the facts
Donald W. Goodwin

Allergy: the facts
R. Davies and S. Ollier

Arthritis and rheumatism: the facts
J. T. Scott

Asthma: the facts
Donald J. Lane and Anthony Storr

Back pain: the facts
Malcolm Jayson

Blindness and visual handicap: the facts
John H. Dobree and Eric Boulter

Blood disorders: the facts
Sheila T. Callender

Breast cancer: the facts
Michael Baum

Cancer: the facts
Sir Ronald Bodley Scott

Childhood diabetes: the facts
J. O. Craig

Contraception: the facts
(second edition) Peter Bromwich and
Tony Parsons

Coronary heart disease: the facts
J. P. Shillingford

Cystic fibrosis: the facts
Ann Harris and Maurice Super

Deafness: the facts
Andrew P. Freeland

Down syndrome: the facts
M. Selikowitz

Eating disorders: the facts
(second edition) S. Abraham and
D. Llewellyn-Jones

Epilepsy: the facts
Anthony Hopkins

Hip replacement: the facts
Kevin Hardinge

Hypothermia: the facts
K. J. Collins

Kidney disease: the facts
(second edition) Stewart Cameron

Liver disease and gallstones: the facts
A. G. Johnson and D. Triger

Lung cancer: the facts
C. J. Williams

Migraine: the facts
F. Clifford Rose and M. Gawel

Miscarriage: the facts
G. C. L. Lachelin

Multiple sclerosis: the facts
(second edition) Bryan Matthews

Parkinson's disease: the facts
(second edition) Gerald Stern and
Andrew Lees

Phobia: the facts
Donald W. Goodwin

Rabies: the facts
(second edition) Colin Kaplan,
G. S. Turner, and D. A. Warrell

Schizophrenia: the facts
Ming Tsuang

Sexually transmitted disease: the facts
David Barlow

Stroke: the facts
F. Clifford Rose and R. Capildeo

Thyroid disease: the facts
R. I. S. Bayliss

Head Injury
THE FACTS

A guide for families and care-givers

Dorothy Gronwall and Philip Wrightson
Auckland Hospital,
Auckland, New Zealand

Peter Waddell
Christchurch Hospital,
Christchurch, New Zealand

Oxford New York Tokyo
OXFORD UNIVERSITY PRESS
1990

Oxford University Press, Walton Street, Oxford OX2 6DP
Oxford New York Toronto
Delhi Bombay Calcutta Madras Karachi
Petaling Jaya Singapore Hong Kong Tokyo
Nairobi Dar es Salaam Cape Town
Melbourne Auckland
and associated companies in
Berlin Ibadan

Oxford is a trade mark of Oxford University Press

Published in the United States
by Oxford University Press, New York

British Library Cataloguing in Publication Data
Gronwall, D.
Head injury : the facts : a guide for families and care-
givers. - (Facts).
1. Head injured patients. 2. Rehabilitation
I. Title II. Wrightson, P. III. Waddell, P. IV. Series
362.19751
ISBN 0-19-261923-3
ISBN 0-19-261922-5 pbk

Library of Congress Cataloging in Publication Data
Gronwall, D. M. A.
Head injury : the facts / Dorothy Gronwall and Philip Wrightson,
Peter Waddell.
(Oxford medical publications)
Includes bibliographical references.
1. Brain—Wounds and injuries. 2. Brain—Wounds and injuries—
Patients—Rehabilitation. I. Wrightson, Philip. II. Waddell,
Peter. III. Title. IV. Series.
[DNLM: 1. Brain Injuries. WL 354 G876h]
RD594.G69 1990 617.4'81044—dc20 90-7050
ISBN 0-19-261923-3
ISBN 0-19-261922-5 (pbk.)

Typeset by Downdell Limited, Oxford
Printed in Great Britain by
Biddles Ltd, Guildford and King's Lynn

Foreword

This is the book which thoughtful clinicians who work with head-injured patients and the patients' families and friends have been waiting for. It comes from the experiences and concerns of authors who are intensively involved with head-injured patients: as scientists trying to understand the nature of the mental and behavioural disturbances which can follow head injury; as clinicians responsible for evaluating and treating these disturbances; and as care-givers who know well the frustrations, disappointments, confusion, and anxiety which are the everyday lot of so many of these patients and their families.

Until very recently the psychological ramifications of head trauma had been largely overlooked, and they were therefore unknown to almost everybody including the patients and the people close to them. Most people suffering a residual compromise of mental efficiency following an accident with minimal or no loss of consciousness attributed their problems to psychological causes; their physicians often dismissed these patients as neurotic, compensation-seekers, or both. Misinterpretation of the more profound behavioural and emotional alterations in severely injured people has also been common. Many of these head-injured people have been dismissed by their families, doctors, and themselves as unmotivated and irresponsible, or have ended up in psychiatric facilities carrying one or another—often several—awesome diagnoses. Only patients with obvious crippling or other physical alteration were likely to have the permanent neuropsychological residuals of their brain injuries recognized, although even then higher mental dysfunctions were often ignored or misinterpreted.

As the misdiagnosed patients have suffered from neglect, bewilderment, and despair, families lacking knowledge about their head-injured patient have suffered too. Many families have gone through a progression of torments that begins with puzzlement and then confusion as the patient no longer responds in familiar and appropriate ways. Frustration and anxiety arise as the uninformed family members discover that their efforts to help the patient are ineffective, and may even make the situation worse. Many family members feel shame and guilt at what they believe are their failures to cope with the patient's problem behaviours. Depression is almost inevitable. Disruption of once solid family relationships is not an infrequent occurrence which further compounds their misery.

It has only been in recent years, as the vicissitudes of head-trauma victims have become known, that there has been a dawning awareness of the profound interdependence between head-injured patients and their families: how the patient can affect the family, what the family can do for the patient. Until now, this information has not been generally available.

Head Injury provides the information family members need, for their own well-being and that of their head-injured patient, by taking the reader from the patient's arrival in an emergency room through typical hospital and post-hospital experiences, emphasizing all the while what the family should know and what family members can do at each stage of the patient's course. More than a manual for patients' families, this book should be required reading for every professional who works with head-injured patients to ensure that they have a practical appreciation of their patients' behaviour and emotions, and sensitivity to the feelings and needs of their patients' families.

Muriel D. Lezak

Acknowledgements

We are grateful for the support of the Medical Research Council of New Zealand and of the New Zealand Neurological Foundation for funding the research of the two senior authors into the effects of head injury; this has allowed us to build up the experience which we have and to gain the basic knowledge which we needed to write this book.

Preface

Will my son make a full recovery? When will he be better? Why does my wife still get so tired when the accident was almost a year ago? When will dad get back to work? Why have our daughter's friends stopped coming to see her?

We have each been asked these and similar questions many many times. This book was written for all those families and friends who want answers about head injury and its effects. It is also written for the teachers and employers and the many people who are involved with return to school, work or family life after head injury. We have tried to anticipate the problems that families may have at each stage of recovery, and to suggest ways of coping with them.

It is a book written in non-technical language which gives practical advice based on our many years of experience in head-injury rehabilitation. It is a reflection of what families have taught us, and of what we have learned from those we have worked with. Do not expect to find detailed discussions of anatomy, physiology, or brain function, because this book deals with the problems that people face in everyday life.

We have answered as many questions as possible. After reading the book we believe that you will have more questions of your own. Hopefully you will now have a better idea of where to go and who to ask.

The majority of people who have head injuries are male, and for this reason we have used the pronouns 'he' and 'him' throughout the book. It avoids the cumbersome 'he or she' or 's/he' which attempts at using a non-sexist style seem to produce. Head injury affects people in similar ways, regardless of sex, and we trust that you will read the book with this in mind.

The tragic lack of appropriate rehabilitation facilities for survivors of head trauma is unfortunately seen all over the world. There are some signs that this is changing, and this change has come about because of the demands of concerned families. We hope that this book will assist you to bring about the changes that you need.

New Zealand   D.G.
1990   P.W.
                                                                                      P.W.

Contents

1. Introduction

The twentieth century is the age of the automobile and the age of speed. It is also the age of the road toll. Each year in developed countries about 20 people of each 100 000 die in road accidents. However horrendous this death toll may be, it is only part of the picture. The hidden road toll, the effect on the drivers, passengers, and pedestrians who suffer head injuries but survive with disability, is as great. There are in addition head injuries from other sorts of accident; in sport, industry, and from violence on the streets.

Statistics from North America, the United Kingdom, and Australasia agree that from every 100 000 people some 200–300 will be admitted to hospital every year because of a head injury. Most of these cases will be due to traffic accidents, and most will be young men in their late teens or early twenties. This is only part of the picture: for each person admitted to hospital two or three will be treated in Casualty Departments or by their family doctors. Although these people have not had life-threatening head injuries, many can have their lives shattered for months or years.

To put the statistics in perspective, in New Zealand with its small population of 3 300 000 there are almost 200 people admitted to hospital each week with head injury, and another 400 are treated but not admitted to hospital. This again is only part of the picture because for each new head injury there are many other people affected. Head injuries involve the family also.

This book has been written for families who have a head-injured member, for people with an injured partner or an injured friend, and especially for all those who, because of circumstances, have taken on the role of care-givers. We have not addressed the book directly to the person who has had the head injury, because the injury will have affected the ability to cope with working through the book. Concentration is invariably impaired following head injury, as is the ability to remember new material. However, we hope that those who have made sufficient recovery from head injury to read this book will find that the information which we have given helps them to understand the injury and its effects. Except where we are specifically talking about women, we have referred to the head-injured person as 'he' for convenience, because most head injury cases are male.

Over the past fifteen years there has been a surge of interest in the problem of head injury. Improved medical techniques have meant that many more people are surviving injuries which in the past would have been fatal. Many articles have been written about the effects of head injury and its treatment but most of the articles are by professionals and written for professionals. The articles appear in scientific journals: you are unlikely to have had access to the articles, which may not be helpful to you in any case. Yet families desperately want to know and understand what happens when one of them suffers a head injury. Time and again, as professionals working in the field of head-injury rehabilitation, we have been asked by families and friends where they can find a book to explain about the head injury. We have not been able to satisfy them in finding a source of information which is comprehensive yet not medical or technical. We hope that this book will fill the gap.

HOW THIS BOOK IS ORGANIZED

The next chapter looks at the mechanics of head injury, and explains how particular parts of the brain become damaged. Chapter 3 covers the period in hospital. The different kinds of hospital treatment and procedures are described, and the sort of information these techniques can and cannot give is explained. Chapter 3 also describes the roles of the different members of the hospital staff and what part each plays in the treatment of the head-injured person.

The remaining chapters talk about the period after he leaves hospital. Head injury is usually a long-term problem, and the emphasis which this book puts on the time after the spell in hospital reflects this. Many of the problems that result from a head injury often only become evident after the head-injured person leaves hospital.

Chapter 4 discusses the practical issues of the post-hospital period. Where will he go? Who will look after him? What treatment will he get, and where? Family involvement and support is a big help to him during the time in hospital. After leaving hospital family involvement and support becomes vital. Usually families are enthusiastic to do as much as they can to help, but often because they are not aware of what is available many do not ask for assistance which they could get. Chapter 4 points out the importance of receiving the financial and other assistance which you are entitled to. Coping with the care of a head-injured person can be a long-term full-time job. Trying to cope with the extra chores that must be done, and with the extra expense that will be involved on an income that is often reduced because of his accident, makes this job even more difficult.

Chapter 5 is the largest and probably the most important in the book. This chapter covers the effect of head injury on emotions and thinking, on how the head-injured person behaves. Most people, even those with quite minor injuries, can have some or all of the problems that are described. This chapter is relevant to everyone, regardless of the type of accident their friend, relative, or partner has had.

Chapter 6 is rather different, covering some special problems that only a proportion of people will have. Some people, for a while, are paralysed down one side of their body after a head injury. Some have difficulty understanding what is said to them, or have trouble talking. Some may have fits or blackouts. Chapter 6 explains why these things happen, and what families can do to cope with them.

Chapter 7 describes the special problems faced by different age groups. It also covers the different (and difficult) problems that head injury can cause when the accident victim is a parent or a partner. Although most head-injured cases are young adult males, accidents can happen to anyone and at any age. The effects of head injury will be similar regardless of the age at which they happen, but these effects pose different problems when they happen at different stages of life. In the first few years of infancy and early childhood, for example, an enormous amount of learning takes place. To learn well you need to have a memory that works well. But head injury almost invariably interferes with how well the memory system will work. So the two-year-old after an accident may take longer to reach some developmental milestones.

Chapter 8 deals with the subject of how long the problems will last. One of the most frustrating things that families have to face is not being able to plan for the future. How long will it be before the head-injured person is able to look after himself again? Will he ever get back to the life he had before the accident? Should his mother give up the career that she may have carved for herself after her children grew up? Should she take leave of absence? You will not find the answers to these questions in this chapter, but we hope that you will understand why they are such difficult questions to answer.

Even if no one can tell you exactly how long it will be before your head-injured relative will be well enough to think about going back to work or to school, in most cases the time will come eventually. Chapter 9 talks about this time, and how the change should be made. It is very important that employers or teachers understand that the person who has had a head injury will get tired more quickly and that he will be more easily distracted. This chapter is therefore addressed to employers and teachers as well as to the people closely involved in caring for him. However, it is important to remember that family support is equally if not more necessary during the gradual shift back to work.

A few head-injured people will never resume employment, and Chapter 10 examines the long-term adjustment that the victim and his family have to make. There are many sorts of loss after severe head injury. There are the obvious losses of physical and mental functions, and the loss of self-esteem and of independence which result. There are the losses of relationships and social life, as well as the loss of careers. Chapter 10 discusses these losses, and suggests how families and head-injured persons can cope with adjusting to permanent disability.

Chapter 11 looks at the future, at the resources which, in an ideal world, should be provided for the head-injured person. It is aimed at those who have the responsibility for the management of the head injured person, and suggests some steps which can be taken to make sure that services are provided. At the end of this chapter there are some suggestions for further reading.

Finally, we have included two appendices. Appendix A is an explanation of many of the technical terms that are used when talking about head injury. Not all these terms have been used in this book, but they are likely to come up when you are talking with doctors or rehabilitation therapists. This appendix should help you to make sense of what has been said or written. Appendix B gives contact addresses of organizations which have been set up to provide support for people who have a relative or friend who has been involved in a head-injury accident. There are three sections in this appendix; for Australasia, for the United Kingdom, and for the United States of America. We believe that it will be helpful for you to have access to the addresses of contact agencies for overseas countries as well as for your own, as there may be cases where a friend or relative has had the injury away from home.

HOW TO USE THIS BOOK

We have aimed to make it as easy as possible for you to find information about any particular problem as it arises. You will find headings in the chapters, and the page numbers of each of these headings are shown in the contents. You may be reading this book for the first time while you are sitting beside your relative in Critical Care, or you may be reading it for the first time many months after the accident. In either case you will be asking for solutions, or at least explanations. The headings are designed to allow you to get directly to the information that you need, now, when you need it. We know, because the care-givers that we have worked with over the years have told us so, that you will want to know everything that you can about head injury. We suspect that you will read this book right through, even though, at any one time, some of the sections will not apply to your case.

CASE HISTORIES

This book includes three case histories which illustrate and summarize many of the points which we cover. The Introduction seems to be as good a place as any to introduce the three cases that we have selected to help you understand head injuries. Names and personal details have been changed to protect the identities of the patients.

Michael—aged 19 years

The accident happened when Michael lost control of his motorcycle on a bend and crashed into a tree. Michael was a university student, living away from home in a student flat. He had been in a reasonably long-term (but not live-in) relationship with his current girl friend, but there had been some problems with this before the accident.

Michael's parents are divorced and live separately, but Michael has maintained contact with both. He has been closest to his mother, who has his 16-year-old sister living with her. There is one other child, an older brother, who lives and works in the town where Michael was at university. Michael has numerous aunts, uncles, and cousins of his own age, who all live in his home town. Although his mother has always been supportive, both she and his father have been concerned about Michael's life-style; they have not approved of his friends, and worry about his abuse of alcohol and soft drugs.

We shall meet Michael again in Chapters 3, 4, 5, 6, 7, 8, and 9.

Mary—aged 8 years

Mary is an eight-year-old schoolgirl who fell onto concrete from a climbing frame in her neighbourhood playground. She has two younger siblings, a six-year-old sister and a four-year-old brother.

Mary has always been a good athlete, and she has done well at sports activities. She loves horse riding and gymnastics, and she is also a good all-rounder. Mary has done well at school, especially since at the age of six years six months she was given an intensive period of remedial teaching for reading delay.

We shall meet Mary again in Chapters 4, 5, 6, 7, 8, and 9.

Arnold—aged 48 years

Arnold is a self-employed business man who had his head injury when the car he was driving collided with a power pole. (As a result of this accident he is waiting for a court hearing to decide if he should be charged with driving while under the influence of alcohol.) Arnold separated from his wife 10 years ago, and has two daughters aged 17 and 21 years old. For the past three years he has had a fairly casual relationship with a girl friend from his single days.

Previously a teacher, Arnold has for the past seven years run a successful restaurant business. Recently he expanded his interests into real estate, and bought some land with options to build: the options run out in 18 months. Arnold bought his present home a year ago, and has major financial commitments, including alimony payments which he has always kept up.

We shall meet Arnold again in Chapters 4, 5, 6, 7, 8, and 9.

2. What happens in a head injury

In this chapter we will try to explain the ways in which the brain may be damaged in an accident, and the effects of this damage. We have found that most families and injured people want to know more about this and that it seems to help them, both in the early days after the accident and in dealing with the problems that come later. You should remember that we are describing a wide range of possibilities, and that the person you are concerned with may have been affected in only one or two of the ways we will be talking about. If you are in doubt about anything, or if what we say worries you, talk it over with the doctor who has been your contact at the hospital or clinic, or with your family doctor.

THE SORTS OF HEAD INJURY

A head injury sets off a train of events. It can help to think of these events in three stages, beginning with the 'first injury', the direct effect of the accident. After this, within an hour or two, the 'second injury' can follow, and in the first day or two the 'third injury'. Each of these injuries can have a decisive effect on the quality of recovery and the success of rehabilitation.

The 'first injury'

> **Three sorts of first injury**
> Closed
> Open
> Crush

Closed head injury
The commonest way the brain can be injured is by 'acceleration', which usually produces a 'closed head injury', called this because there is

usually no break of the skin or an open wound. This happens when the head suddenly changes its motion. Examples are the sudden stop when a car runs into a brick wall (deceleration), or when one car runs into another from behind at the traffic lights (acceleration). Another example is the sudden roll of the head with a knock-out punch to the jaw (rotation).

As the head is accelerated, decelerated, or rotated the brain is forced to follow the movement of the skull, and as the brain is soft and jelly-like it gets twisted and distorted in the process. The brain is made up of billions of nerve fibres, which lead from one part of the brain to the other, and as the twisting occurs these fibres are stretched and damaged. Quite mild injuries of this sort are important because of the way that the damage is spread widely throughout the brain.

The arteries and veins which run through the brain are torn and blood leaks from them, making a bruise which is very like one anywhere else in the body.

Also, because there is room for the brain to move a little inside the skull, with the acceleration it slides on the inner surface of the bone. This surface has ridges and sharp edges which cause the surface of the brain to be bumped and bruised, resulting in more damage.

Penetrating head injury

The second sort of 'first injury' is the 'penetrating' or 'open' injury. In this type of injury the scalp is cut through, the bone of the skull beneath it can be broken up, and the brain exposed and damaged. The causes of injury range from collisions with the sharp edge of a stone curb, a motor cycle brake lever, a length of reinforcing steel, or being hit by a bullet. Unfortunately the open injury is often accompanied by an acceleration type injury as well. If this is not the case, however, the brain area away from the immediate area of the injury is likely to be undamaged, and in the long term there may be very little disability in spite of what seems at the time to be a frightening injury.

Crushing head injury

The third type of 'first injury' is the 'crushing' injury: the head may be caught between a boat and the wharf or under the wheel of a car. This is the least common sort of injury: often the important damage is not to the brain itself but to the base of the skull and the nerves that run out through it, and there may be no loss of consciousness.

In all types of 'first injury' almost every time what really matters is the injury to the brain itself. The scalp can be torn and the bone of the skull can be broken or parts of it lost, but if there is any long-term disability it will be because of damage to the brain underneath.

The second accident

Many serious injuries result from high-speed car accidents. The head is damaged when the first collision occurs, but then the victim may be flung out of the car and strike his head again, perhaps even several times, and also incur other injuries. This is a very important cause of multiple major injuries, and it must be emphasized that efficient seat belts will stop this happening.

The 'first injury'—occurs in the first 2 seconds

Brain accelerated, decelerated, or rotated

Nerve fibres stretched

Arteries and veins torn

With or without an open wound

Note: Sometimes there is a second accident

Seatbelts stop the second accident

The 'first injury' to the brain as we have described it takes place within a second. In this short time much of the fate of the victim is decided. Not all of it, however, because in many people there are at least two further injuries.

The 'second injury'

Most accidents happen in the worst surroundings; at night, in the rain, away from expert help. The victim can be crushed into the twisted body of his car, with his face buried in the seat. His breathing is often blocked with vomited food, or blood from an injury to his nose or face. Air cannot get to the lungs and the result is that the amount of oxygen in the blood becomes much less than it should be. The brain is then starved of oxygen, which kills its cells and makes the damage from the first injury worse.

Injuries to other parts of the body are common in road accidents like this, and often a great deal of blood is lost. This lowers the blood pressure below normal limits and reduces the supply of blood, and therefore oxygen, to the brain, thus increasing the brain damage.

Understanding this chain of events has led to great improvements in the way ambulance and rescue services operate. The first thing they will do at the scene of the accident will be to make sure that breathing is free and easy, then they will set up an urgent transfusion to replace the blood lost and to bring the blood pressure back to normal. By doing this the brain is protected and the journey to hospital is made safe with further injury prevented.

The 'second injury'—occurs in the first hour

Low blood pressure reduces supply of blood, and therefore oxygen, to the brain

---

The 'third injury'

The injuries we have described up to now have occurred in the first second after the accident and in the first hour. The 'third injury' can occur any time after this, usually in the next two or three days, but sometimes up to months later. There are several forms it can take.

Bruising and swelling of the brain

When it is damaged at the first impact the brain reacts to injury in the same way as the rest of the body does, by bruising; the brain swells because body fluids and blood leak out into it. The effect is more important than in other parts of the body because the brain is enclosed tightly in the unyielding skull. Even slight swelling squeezes the brain, so that blood has difficulty in circulating through it. In severe cases the pressure in the brain can become so high that the blood circulation in the brain stops entirely, and the brain then dies.

The pressure inside the head (you may hear it called the 'intracranial pressure' or 'ICP') is therefore something of great importance. The medical team needs to know what it is when they are planning treatment, and much of what they do will be designed to keep it at a safe level. As we will see in Chapter 3, sometimes intracranial pressure is measured continuously and displayed on one of the 'monitor' screens around the patient in intensive care.

To keep the intracranial pressure down the brain swelling must be kept to a minimum. To do this, the first thing is to make sure that the blood coming to the brain has plenty of oxygen in it and that it is removing waste products like carbon dioxide. The blood pressure must be kept high enough to keep the brain circulation going. Air (perhaps with oxygen added) must flow in and out of the lungs without any obstruction. There must be no coughing or straining, which puts the intracranial pressure up and starts fresh bleeding in damaged areas of the brain. Finally, the amount of water and salt in the body must be kept at the right level to reduce the flow of tissue fluid into the brain. Frequent blood tests will be done to make sure of this, and the amount of water given will be strictly controlled.

Blood clots

We have described how at the time of the original injury small veins and arteries are torn and that this results in bruising of the brain. Sometimes larger blood vessels are torn, so that enough blood escapes in one place to form a ball of blood clot which compresses and damages the brain around it. It also increases the intracranial pressure, and if the bleeding does not stop it can push the intracranial pressure over the limit at which it becomes fatal.

These clots are not very common, but they are important. They can occur after quite minor injuries, even when the victim has been knocked out for only a short period and has apparently recovered. This is one of the reasons why even minor injuries are taken seriously by hospital accident departments, and why people are kept under observation until the risk of clots forming is likely to be over. When there is a serious injury the risk is greater, and many of the observations in intensive care are designed to detect them as early as possible. The second reason why blood clots are so important is that if they do occur, they can usually be treated successfully by operation.

In discussing the situation with the family the medical team may refer to where the clot is; this could be in the brain (an intracerebral clot), in the space round the brain (an acute subdural clot), or in the space between the bone and the dura, the thick membrane surrounding the brain (an extradural clot). The exact location really only matters to the surgeon who removes it, and it is probably better not to complicate the issue with further detail.

There is, however, one special case that you should know about and that is the 'chronic subdural haematoma'. This is most often seen in older people and it can follow quite a minor injury. What happens is that a small clot forms between the brain and the dura, not big enough to be detected at first. This slowly grows in size over weeks until it is large enough to cause symptoms of pressure on the brain. Fortunately it can usually be removed by a simple operation, and the results of doing this are good.

Another condition which comes on later with symptoms rather like the chronic subdural haematoma is 'post-traumatic hydrocephalus'. This occurs when the circulation of the fluid round the brain is blocked by the scarring which follows the brain injury. The fluid accumulates within the brain and the intracranial pressure rises. Again this complication can be treated very effectively by a small operation.

The 'third injury'—occurs days or weeks later

A *day or more later*:
brain swelling and bruising
blood clots

A *week or more later*:
chronic subdural haematoma
post-traumatic hydrocephalus

DAMAGE TO THE SKULL

It was said earlier on that it was the damage to the brain itself that was the most important thing about a head injury. This is so, but the skull is often damaged as well and sometimes needs treatment.

Fractures of the vault

The commonest damage, a 'linear fracture', is a crack in the vault of the skull, the rounded dome of the head. This is usually not more than a millimetre or so wide, and it is not of itself important, although of course it does mean that the blow to the head was quite severe and that some of the complications we have mentioned are more likely to occur. It heals quickly, usually with scar tissue rather than bone, and leaves no weakness.

A blow to the vault of the skull can crack the bone and 'dent' it, sometimes pushing a piece of bone far enough in to damage the underlying brain. This 'depressed fracture' may need an operation, not usually a serious one, to replace the fragments and to deal with the damaged brain under them.

Fractures of the forehead, nose, and eye sockets

If a fracture involves the bone of the forehead or the roof of the nose then there may be a hole in the roof of the nose so that the brain fluid (cerebrospinal fluid) leaks out and drips from the nose. The important consequence is that bacteria may get in through the hole and infect the brain, so causing meningitis. In the short term infection can be prevented by giving antibiotics, but unless the leak stops soon of its own accord an operation will be needed to block the hole up and make a permanent repair. This is usually not a serious matter. A similar leak can occur when there is a fracture of the skull which involves the bone round the middle ear; this usually heals of its own accord.

Some severe injuries fracture the bone of the eye sockets and the middle part of the face, as well as the vault of the skull which encloses the brain. This can interfere with the nasal sinuses and alter the alignment of the teeth in the upper jaw. It can be very unsightly and an operation, usually done by a team of neurosurgeons and plastic surgeons, may be needed to correct the deformity.

Fractures with wounds

When there is a penetrating injury the bone of the skull can be damaged. An urgent operation will be needed to clean the wound and get rid of infection, and to close the skin. Sometimes pieces of bone will be missing or too badly damaged to replace. This is not important at the time, and no harm will result. Later, if the gap in the skull is big enough to be a risk, or looks ugly, it can be closed. After several months, when the wound has healed and all chance of infection is gone, a bone graft or a plastic or metal plate can be put in to fill in the hole.

Damage to the skull

Fractures of the vault:
linear fractures: only important because they show there has been
   a significant injury
depressed fractures: bone may need to be lifted   (cont.)

Damage to the skull (cont.)
Fractures of the forehead, nose, and eye sockets:
may cause leaks of cerebrospinal fluid
ugly deformities may need operation

Fractures with wounds:
will need operation to prevent infection
defects in the skull may need to be filled in

LATE EFFECTS OF HEAD INJURY

Multiple head injuries

Many people have more than one head injury. This is especially important for two reasons. Firstly, the brain may become abnormally sensitive to injury. If there is a further accident within a week or two of the first, when the brain is still recovering, there may be a reaction quite out of proportion to the severity of either injury, and which may even be fatal. This is an important reason why sportsmen who have been concussed should not be allowed to play again for at least three or four weeks after the injury.

Secondly, there is the general loss of brain power that follows multiple head injuries. Even if there has been only one injury before, a second injury seems to have much more of an effect than would be expected, and after each further injury the disturbance becomes more marked. Progressive damage can occur with quite minor injuries. Football players after only three or four concussions can begin to show obvious deterioration in their thinking powers. An extreme example is the punch-drunk boxer; it is not necessary for him to have been knocked out a large number of times to produce this condition as he only needs to have taken sufficient punches to the head.

The reason for progressive deterioration is probably that each injury kills some nerve cells, so that the total number available to do the work of the brain is steadily reduced. Eventually the reserve which we all have becomes exhausted. With further injury, or sometimes with the loss of brain cells which occurs with age, there is not enough brain left to do the work asked of it and obvious symptoms appear.

> **Multiple head injuries**
>
> Some brain function is lost with each injury
>
> Multiple minor injuries can cause brain loss, and blows without loss of consciousness can destroy brain cells

Post-traumatic epilepsy

When the brain is damaged, it heals with a scar. As it does this the brain around the damaged area begins to work in an abnormal way. It becomes irritable and unstable, and liable to bursts of uncontrolled activity. The disturbance tends to spread out from the damaged area and involve the rest of the brain, and this produces an epileptic fit. This is most often seen after a severe injury, especially when there has been much bruising or bleeding into the brain, or if the brain has been damaged in an open wound. Sometimes it can follow a minor injury if the injury has resulted in even a small bruise in a particularly sensitive area.

The effect of the injury on brain function

It has been known for a long time that damage to particular areas of the brain is followed by characteristic effects on function. For instance, wounds of the side of the head, half way from front to back (the 'parietal' area), result in weakness of the arm or leg on the opposite side of the body. Damage on the left side of the brain tends to impair speech. Injury to the brain behind the forehead (the 'frontal' area) results in changes in behaviour, and loss of self restraint and insight.

If there is a localized injury to the brain, caused by an open wound or a penetrating injury, only one of these functions may be affected. Most head injuries, however, are closed injuries caused by an acceleration, and many areas of the brain are affected at the same time. Some or even all of the changes described above are likely to be found together, some being more severe than others. Furthermore, whilst wounds or penetrating injuries usually damage just the surface of the brain, in closed injuries the nerve fibres deep in the brain are damaged. These include the central parts of the brain which are vital for keeping us alert, and it is the damage here that results in the most typical symptom of head injury—coma.

Often torn in a deeper injury are the big bundles of nerves which run down from the surface areas of the brain to the centre, the brain stem and the spinal cord, and which control movement and feeling. This results in a characteristic type of paralysis of the arms and legs. The muscles remain tight, the legs are stretched out straight and stiff, and the arms are bent at the elbow—a 'spastic' paralysis. Both legs are often affected and only one arm. When movement eventually returns, it is likely to be awkward and uncoordinated.

The movements of the throat are under the control of the brainstem, and the impairment of speech and swallowing which are so often present after a serious injury are due to damage there. The brain stem is also responsible for body functions which are not under conscious control; breathing, heart beat and blood pressure, and body temperature, and upset of these functions may be one of the factors which determine survival in the early days after the injury.

Many of the effects described above will be visible while the victim is still unconscious or semi-conscious. It will not be until later that the more subtle effects on thinking and personality become obvious. These effects on thinking and personality are partly due to damage in the special areas which we described at the beginning of this section, but they are due more to the widespread tearing of nerve fibres that affects all the working parts of the brain.

Effect on brain function

Visible effects:
coma
loss of power in limbs (often spastic)
impaired speech and swallowing

Hidden effects:
on heart, blood pressure, and breathing (in the early stages)
on thinking and personality (in the later stages)

RECOVERY AFTER INJURY

Although it is not known for certain, it is likely that most of the brain cells which have been damaged will not get back to useful work. The majority of the improvement which is seen after a head injury is due to reorganization of the brain which is undamaged. Using the large reserves of brain function which we all have, functional areas take over from the areas which are no longer functional. Obviously, if these reserves of brain have been reduced by previous injuries, or the natural loss of cells with age, recovery will be less complete.

Recovery therefore is a matter of learning and re-education. It may take a long time, comparable to the years spent in school. Recovery will depend on consistent teaching and patient encouragement, and to be effective it must occupy most of the waking day. On this basis the programme of rehabilitation will need to be planned.

Recovery after injury

The best use should be made of undamaged abilities

Re-education can take as long as education

Rehabilitation is a full-time job

BRAIN DEATH

It is sometimes not possible to overcome the effects of the injury. The cause is almost always that the swelling of the brain and the pressure inside the skull cannot be controlled. As the pressure rises, the circulation of the blood slows and eventually stops. After a few minutes the brain is irreparably damaged. The spinal cord may remain alive for a while, and there may be some automatic reflexes in the limbs, but all other functions stop.

Although it is usually only too obvious when brain death has taken place, because of the need to be absolutely certain most doctors follow a routine of tests, repeated several times at intervals of an hour or two. The simple tests are the important ones. There are no reflexes which require brain function; the pupils of the eyes are widely dilated and do not react to light and there is no effort to breathe even with the maximum stimulation. Other tests can be used to confirm these findings if there is any doubt. The electroencephalogram, which records the electrical activity of the brain, will be absent. X-ray tests can be done to see if there is any circulation of blood to the brain.

When it is certain that there is no longer any chance of recovery of function of the brain, it is usually taken that there is no use to continuing treatment, and if the family agrees the life-support systems can be withdrawn.

If it has been decided that treatment should stop, the family may be asked for their agreement to allow body organs such as the kidneys and heart to be removed for use as transplants. It is very difficult to make decisions at a time like this. There may be good reasons to say no. However, it is worthwhile here reassuring you about two questions which are often asked. Firstly, there is no question of using the organs unless there is absolutely no doubt that there has been brain death. It will not be done until the tests described above have been checked and until an independent medical team is absolutely certain about them. Secondly, there is the question as to whether or not the transplants actually do good. About this there is again no doubt; they are likely to mean the difference between life and death for two or more people.

3. In hospital

The care of someone with a head injury starts with first aid at the site of the accident, it continues with rescue by the ambulance and paramedics, and it is followed through by a team working in the hospital, using all its facilities.

Whether you are the patient or one of his family, if you have not been involved with a hospital before then you may feel very lost and frightened by this large organization, with all its power and prestige. It is a good idea, therefore, to know how a hospital works, who you may meet, and what they do. It is also a good idea to remember that you have very definite rights in this situation, and that the whole organization was set up for your benefit.

To give you the best idea of how it all works we will follow Michael, the young man introduced in Chapter 1 who has had a serious traffic accident, from the crash site to the time he leaves hospital. Afterwards, we will talk about what happens to victims with less serious injuries, and we shall discuss some other special situations.

RESCUE: FIRST AID AND THE AMBULANCE

Michael came off his motorbike and hit a tree. He had a gash in his thigh which bled heavily and he was unconscious. His friend John, who was behind him on another bike, found him. A motorist telephoned for an ambulance, which arrived 15 minutes after the accident.

In Chapter 2 this was called the time of the 'second injury'. The victim may be unable to breathe properly because of the position he is lying in, or because his throat is blocked with blood or vomit. The injured brain does not get enough oxygen, so causing further damage. John tried to get Michael's face and mouth clear of clothes, vomit, and blood as best he could. At the same time he had to be careful not to move Michael too much in case there were other injuries. As an aside, even if you have been sensible and have taken first aid classes, in some situations first aid may not be easy to administer, and no one should feel guilty if they cannot do it.

When the ambulance arrived, it was staffed by paramedics who were

expert in dealing with severe injuries. They started by making sure he
could breathe. They sometimes put a tube down the throat into the windpipe to ensure that the airway is free and unobstructed, but this did not
seem necessary here. They looked after the wound in the thigh to stop it
bleeding during transport to hospital, and saw to some minor injuries.

Another factor in the 'second injury' is loss of blood. If there are
wounds which bleed heavily, or if there is severe bruising, the blood
pressure will fall below normal and the blood supply of the brain will not
be sufficient to supply the brain with the oxygen it needs. For this reason
the paramedics put up a transfusion to replace the blood which Michael
had lost, so bringing the blood pressure up to normal. As blood itself
needs cross matching in the laboratory before it can be used, at the site of
the accident blood substitutes are given.

Michael needed hospitalization as soon as possible. Helicopters can cut
the travelling time down and are often used when the accident has
happened in rough country or away from roads, but the accommodation
for patient and attendants can be cramped. A road ambulance may take a
little longer over the journey, but it may be easier to keep a closer watch
on the patient than in a helicopter.

Paramedics at the scene of the accident will:

Ensure that the victim is breathing
Replace lost blood
Make wounds and fractures safe for transport

REACHING HOSPITAL

As soon as Michael reached hospital the medical team made a complete
examination. The first thing to be seen was that he was deeply unconscious. His breathing, which had been easy before, was now difficult. A
tube was threaded through his nose into his windpipe (an 'endotracheal
tube'), which was connected to a mechanical ventilator to do his
breathing for him. Michael could then be given muscle relaxing drugs to
let him rest quietly without coughing or straining, both of which are bad
for the brain, and so that he did not have to put what energy he had left
into the effort of breathing. When this had been done, the oxygen could

get to his blood, his colour became better, and it was obvious that his general condition had improved.

The rest of his body was then examined, starting with the head, and then looking particularly for injuries to the chest, abdomen, and spine, areas which are often injured in this sort of accident. X-rays of the chest and neck were carried out as a routine. Fortunately in Michael's case there was no sign of damage. The amount of blood that had been lost was assessed. This was more than what could be replaced safely by blood substitutes, so blood was cross matched and a transfusion started.

Essential checks on arrival at hospital
Breathing checked
Blood loss assessed
Head injury checked
Neck, spine, chest, and abdomen examined

All this initial treatment was done at a run, and was completed within 15 minutes of Michael being wheeled through the door. Notice that so far we have said very little about the head injury itself. This may be surprising, but in fact at this stage nothing needs to be done for the head injury except to give the brain the best conditions to recover; a good circulation, plenty of oxygen, and no straining. Now the head injury has to be looked at in more detail.

When Michael first came into the hospital and before the muscle relaxing drugs were given, a very rapid examination of brain function was made. The depth of unconsciousness was recorded as a 'coma score', so that changes could be followed later. His arms and legs were examined to see if they moved when the skin was pinched, and the pupils of the eyes were tested to see how they reacted to light. The amount of information that can be obtained from an unconscious patient is limited, but these simple tests will usually show if there is any serious damage to the function of the brain. In addition, a note was made of bruises and wounds on the head, which can give useful clues to damage inside.

Michael was fortunate because when he was first examined all four limbs moved equally and his pupils reacted normally. Now, two hours or so after the accident, he had come to the stage where the chance of the 'third injury' that we spoke of in Chapter 2 had become important. Pressure could be developing inside the skull, either because of bruising of the brain or because a clot of blood had formed. If Michael had not been so badly injured and if he had remained partially awake then this would have shown by his becoming less conscious, and perhaps by one side of his body becoming weak or paralysed. Because Michael was deeply unconscious, and because he had been given relaxing drugs which abolished movement, these signs were not available, and so the team had to rely on high-technology tests. As soon as possible, X-rays were taken of the head.

High-technology tests

X-rays

Ordinary X-rays show only the bone of the skull, not the brain. It is of course useful to know whether there is a fracture of the skull, or if any fragments of bone have been pushed into the brain, but at this stage what matters is what is happening to the brain itself. The state of the bone is only a rough guide. To show up the brain itself, special X-ray methods are needed, and the one which at the moment replaces all others is the CT scan.

CT scan

The CT ('Computerized Tomographic') scanner can show the soft tissue of the brain itself. It can be seen whether it is bruised or swollen, and if there is a blood clot forming. This is just the information which we need.

Michael was taken to the CT scanner with his transfusion lines and ventilator attached. The examination showed that there was a clot of blood between the bone of the skull and the outer covering of the brain (the 'dura mater') just above his left ear, with much pressure on the brain. This had to be removed and a neurosurgical operation was needed.

Clues to what is happening in the brain

CT scans:	give the most complete picture
Skull X-rays *Bruises, wounds* }	provide some information
Depth of coma *Movement* }	provide information only in the absence of relaxing drugs

---

The people involved up to now

The team which has worked on Michael up to now is called the Intensive Care team, sometimes the Critical Care or the Trauma team. They are the experts in dealing with the severely injured whose need is to be kept alive and protected from the effects of their multiple injuries. When problems arise in special fields, the Intensive Care team will call on other experts; orthopaedic (bone and joint) surgeons for fractures, abdominal or chest surgeons for injuries to the trunk, and neurosurgeons for the head.

One of the team rang Michael's family as soon as the ambulance brought him in, and talked with them as soon as they arrived at the Accident Department. He told them that Michael's injuries were serious, and that they would have to prepare themselves for the possibility that he might not survive. More than this he was unable to say, and they had to accept that at this stage. There was just not enough information to give them any further guide.

It is important for families to realize that right from the beginning, and for weeks to come, it will only be possible for the doctors to give them an uncertain guess about what the future holds. The doctors can tell that an injury is a severe one, or not so severe. They know that a certain percentage of people with severe injuries will die, that some will recover but with a handicap, and that others will do well. Saying that one particular patient, your Michael, will do this or that can only be a guess guided by these probabilities. It is understandable that families desperately want to know what is going to happen, but they need to realize that there is no definite answer for an honest doctor to give. The hard news is that the family must wait and see.

Michael's parents asked if they might see their son. They felt that it was good for them to be with Michael for a moment, even if he was deeply unconscious and surrounded by tubes, machines, and a team working flat out. Some people would find this distressing and prefer to stay away; there should be no guilt in this.

After Michael's parents had seen their son, he was taken to the X-ray department for the CT scan. When it was known that an operation was needed, the neurosurgeon talked to Michael's parents to tell them what the situation was and what he thought was needed.

When Michael was first brought in to hospital the situation was critical. Every moment counted, and there was no time to find the family, tell them what ought to be done, and to get permission to do it. Treatment had to go ahead in good faith. There is now not quite so much urgency, and before operating on Michael there is a little time for discussion with the family and to ask for their consent. The situation and the risks need to be explained, both those of going ahead and of doing nothing. However fully and sympathetically the situation is explained, family may feel that they have little say in the matter. As the decisions are forced on the team by the nature of the injury, there is probably no way round this, but the staff should be full and open about the situation and answer questions patiently. The family are entitled to expect this. The family should also try to realize that although the staff are professionals meeting similar situations every day, they still become emotionally involved and need support and recognition if they are to do their job well.

Staff need to explain the situation:

as soon as possible
in as much detail as possible
as often as asked

Family need to realize:

there are no certainties, only probabilities
professionals are human

SURGERY

Brain operations are unfamiliar and the thought of them often distresses people. In fact the operations needed for head injuries are usually straightforward and themselves involve little risk. The real cause for anxiety is the condition which made them necessary, and how much damage it has already done. This will usually only become apparent much later on, when consciousness has returned and it can be seen how the brain is functioning.

In Michael's case, the blood clot which was pressing on his brain was removed by cutting a trapdoor in the bone of the skull exactly over the clot (the CT scan had shown the place) and then by washing the clot away. The bone, which was put back and fastened in place, had healed firmly by three or four weeks and left no weakness.

The other sort of operation which is sometimes needed for head injuries is one to repair open wounds. These can look very frightening, especially if the brain is showing in them. This situation can usually be dealt with quite easily and successfully, often with little long-term disability.

INTENSIVE CARE

Whether an operation is needed or not, people with severe head injuries will need to be looked after in Intensive Care for a time. Their whole system has been upset, blood has been lost, and, apart from the head, other parts of the body have been damaged by the accident itself, and by the low blood pressure and lack of oxygen that so often follows. The changes in the condition of the victim have to be watched very carefully and treatment needs adjusting from hour to hour. The assisted breathing with the ventilator that was started in the Accident Department is an important part of this programme of care, and it will need to be continued for several days so that the head has the best chance of improving.

Intensive Care monitoring

In order to monitor all these factors means that Michael has to be connected with tubes and wires to several machines, each with its own TV monitor. The action of his heart shows continually on the electrocardiogram, and often on the same screen his blood pressure is recorded, taken by putting a fine tube in a small artery in his ankle or arm. Sometimes the pressure inside the head is measured continuously with a lead from inside the skull, and this will show on another screen. To feed Michael and give him the medication he needs, a drip transfusion is put into a vein in his arm. Lastly, there are the controls of the ventilator, the number of breaths a minute and how deep they are, which have to be managed to keep the pressure of oxygen and carbon dioxide in the blood at the correct levels. Other tests will be done as they are needed. Blood will be examined regularly. CT scans will be repeated to check whether there has been any further brain swelling or if more clots develop.

EEG

Tests of the electrical function of the brain are sometimes used. In the electroencephalogram (EEG) the small electric currents, which come from the action of the brain, are picked up by wires attached to the scalp and recorded on paper. This can help to tell how the brain is working and if function is recovering.

SEPs

Another test is measurement of the 'Sensory Evoked Potentials' (SEPs). If a nerve in the arm or leg is stimulated by a small electric current, the EEG will change. The time it takes to change is increased when the deep parts of the brain (the 'brain stem') are damaged. The first results will give an idea of how bad the damage is, and repeated tests show if recovery is taking place. These tests are useful in expert hands, but they are not essential to good care and they are only done in large hospitals with specialist neurological units.

These methods of looking after people who have been severely injured have only developed in the last 20 years or so, and a new sort of medical specialist, the 'intensivist' that we mentioned before, has developed to manage them. The new approach to accident care has resulted in an enormous increase in the number of lives saved.

Mechanical ventilation

One of the difficult decisions that has to be made is how long to use the ventilator for. The quiet breathing, the prevention of coughing and straining, and the right amount of oxygen and carbon dioxide in the blood create the best conditions for healing the brain. The ventilator may also be needed to manage chest or other injuries. It does have its disadvantages, however, and the intensivists will want to dispense with it as soon as it is safe to do so. When things seem to be settling they will weigh up the pros and cons, and if they think that the conditions are right they will start to allow normal breathing, and see if it is adequate. Sometimes it turns out to be too early, and ventilation has to be continued for another day or two until another attempt can be made to discontinue it.

If ventilation has to be continued for more than three or four days the tube may start to irritate the windpipe and perhaps damage it. It may be best then to put in a 'tracheostomy' tube. At a small operation, usually with a local anaesthetic, the windpipe is opened through an incision in the neck just below the 'Adam's apple' and a plastic tube threaded in. The ventilator is then connected to this. When the ventilator is no longer needed the tube can be used for normal breathing for a while until it is certain that there is no obstruction to the airway. Eventually the tube can be removed, and after a few days the hole in the neck will heal by itself.

Fluids and feeding

The other change as things improve is in the method of feeding. To begin with all the fluid and food that Michael needed had to be given by transfusion. After a day or two, as his condition became more stable, a fine tube could be passed down his throat into his stomach (a 'nasogastric tube'). Liquid food, and later puréed meals, were given through this.

Special nursing care

People who lie unconscious need special nursing care. Pressure on the skin has to be avoided. Joints will get stiff if they are not moved regularly. Splints for fractures of limbs need adjustment. Nurses and physiotherapists will be constantly attending to this.

All the measures taken were necessary to keep Michael alive. A day after the operation another CT scan was done, which showed that the brain had settled down well after the clot had been removed. It was not yet possible to tell how his brain was working because of the relaxing drugs and sedation. However, he seemed to be ready to breathe on his own and it was possible to discontinue the ventilator. He was still unconscious, but he would move his arms and legs if stimulated and there did not seem to be any paralysis.

In another couple of days Michael began to open his eyes when he was spoken to, and to move around a little in his bed. He had not yet tried to swallow, and feeding was continued by his nasogastric tube. His condition was stable, he no longer needed life support, and he was ready to pass on to the next stage.

Intensive care: around the clock

Checking heart, blood pressure
Controlling breathing
Controlling fluids and food
Testing brain function
Waiting for the patient to take over his own body management

HEAD-INJURY WARD

At the next stage the patient is taken to the 'Head-Injury Ward', but its name and where it fits into the rest of the hospital will vary from place to place. In large hospitals it may be the neurosurgical ward, in smaller ones a general surgical ward which will take all sorts of cases. It could be a special unit for head-injury care and rehabilitation, although these are not common yet. Who is in charge will vary, therefore, but in general there will be a senior doctor with responsibility for the overall medical care, and a charge nurse who runs the ward. There will be junior doctors, in the British system called registrars and house surgeons (residents and interns in North America), and nurses responsible to the charge nurse. There will also be people expert in other forms of treatment: physiotherapists (PTs) who will look after muscles and joints; occupational therapists (OTs) who will help to restore the everyday activities of living; speech therapists, dieticians, and psychologists. All these people will come into contact with Michael and have an effect on his recovery.

One of the big problems which Michael's family will have is knowing who to go to for information, and how to sort out what the advice from the various team members adds up to. The larger units, accustomed to head-injured victims and their families, will have worked this out. Regular briefing sessions should be arranged so that the family knows exactly what is happening, and so that the members of the team can pass on their instructions directly. Family will often be tempted to try to get information about progress outside these sessions, and to ask the nurse at the bedside or a house surgeon met casually in the corridor how things are going. The nurse and the doctor will be tempted to help, but they may not have the up-to-date answers, and they may say something which ends up in misunderstanding and chaos. It is much the wisest course only to look for important information from the person in charge, or from someone nominated by him.

Smaller units may not have the process as well organized as this. You are again strongly recommended to insist on seeing the person ultimately responsible for care, and to ask this person what you need to know. It should be possible to make a regular appointment to do this.

> **Staff need to arrange regular communication:**
> give as much information as possible
> as often as asked
> by the same person each time, if at all possible

Let us now return to Michael, who had reached the stage when he was responding to his family with simple words, and moving around on his own. He soon began to eat a little and it was safe to remove the nasogastric tube; at this stage in some units X-ray tests are done to make sure that the swallowing mechanism has recovered properly. The physiotherapists were helping him to get back his strength; the occupational therapists were teaching him to look after himself, and to wash and dress. He was encouraged to do anything which would help to get his skills back; puzzles, hobbies, music, or games. At first he had some problems with finding the right words; this is often found in victims with some damage to the left side of the brain, and he needed the help of the speech therapists.

We mentioned previously that the members of the medical team passed on their instructions to the family. These instructions, and carrying them out, become vital at this stage. There are never enough staff to give all the treatment which is needed, and family will have to do a great deal to back up the treatment of the professionals; of course, there are also things which only the family can do, such as reminding him of his life before the accident, and re-introducing him to his old world. Family are entitled to ask what the reason for each recommendation is. Sometimes the family may not feel themselves that it is the right thing to do. If this is the case they should talk it out with the staff. The family should never agree to one thing and do another; this can do untold harm to the patient, the one person who really matters.

A fortnight after going to the head-injury ward Michael was up and walking around. He was not yet behaving normally, and he had a number of problems with mental function and behaviour which are described in other parts of this book. As he was able to do more, he began to go on expeditions out of hospital with his family, first for an hour or two, then overnight, and then for weekends. He no longer needed the sort of care which is given in an acute ward of a hospital, and he could now move on to the next stage of his recovery. This transition, and the problems it raises, are described in the next chapter.

Some people who have had head injuries are less fortunate than Michael. Their brains have been more severely damaged. Coma may last for months. Recovery is agonizingly slow, or may seem to stop when there are still severe disabilities. The stress on families becomes severe. This situation is discussed in the following chapters.

The Head-Injury Ward

Returns the patient to:
independent feeding
independent moving
self care
ability to communicate
the family

MODERATELY SEVERE HEAD INJURIES

Many people have head injuries which need treatment in hospital, but the injuries are not bad enough to need the intensive care which we have described. Usually the victim will have been seen in the accident department of the hospital, and from there admitted to a ward, probably the Head-Injury Ward we described above. The patient may already be awake when he gets to the ward, or he may be semi-conscious and remain in that state for a day or two. His progress will be like Michael's, but probably much faster, and he will receive much the same treatment.

There are two main considerations while the patient is in hospital. After even quite mild injuries complications can occur—the 'third injury' that we described before. These must be recognized at once and treated. A large part of the care that is given will therefore consist of regular observations and tests such as CT scans.

Some victims in the early stages will require the same sort of care that was given to the severe injuries. They will need nursing care to watch for the onset of complications, for feeding, and for toileting. As happens with any sort of head injury, they may become restless, confused, or aggressive, requiring special management. Later, problems with movement and balance, thinking, and behaviour can become evident, and physiotherapists, occupational therapists, speech therapists, and psychologists may be involved.

The hospital staff that the family will have to deal with have been described above, and there should be the same care in making sure that family get reliable information.

It is important that a patient of this group is reviewed at a set time after the injury, either at a hospital clinic or by a family doctor or specialist. Even the victim who seems to recover quickly may later find that he has persisting problems. These are discussed in Chapter 5.

Less severe injuries

Recover more quickly but:
they have the same risks
they need the same precautions
they may leave problems of thinking and behaviour when
 recovery seems complete
the family still needs to be kept informed

MILD HEAD INJURIES

For every person who is admitted to hospital after a head injury three or more will be seen in the accident department and then allowed to go home. Many of these will have recovered completely by the time they get to hospital, and they have attended just to be checked. Some will have been semi-conscious or confused but have recovered after an hour or two. Some will have needed to have cuts on their scalp cleaned and stitched.

The importance of a hospital visit for these people, apart from the care of cuts and other minor injuries, is to deal with the risk of the 'third injury', for these complications can follow even minor head injury. Because of the seriousness of this problem hospitals have very strict rules to sort out those who can safely be allowed to go home. They vary a little from place to place, but the rules are generally along these lines:

1. People who are safe to go home must be free from any sign of complication, thinking clearly with normal memory, with good balance, and with only minor headache.

2. There must not be any sign of a skull fracture. The fracture itself does not matter, but complications are perhaps thirty times more

common in people who have one. Some hospitals make it a rule to X-ray everyone, but probably this is unnecessary and wasteful, and X-rays need only to be carried out if there is a definite indication that a fracture might be present.

3. There must be someone to look after them when they get home.

Many hospitals make special rules for children and old people, who sometimes have particular risks of complications.

Remember!

You have a right to competent and compassionate treatment and
   to choice
You have a right to information
The person you ask can only give you probabilities
Head injuries take a long time to heal

---

4. Leaving hospital—what happens now?

After the first dreadful days or weeks when you did not know whether your friend or relative was going to live or die, having him well enough to leave hospital became your goal. You spent as much time as possible at the bedside with him, even when he was unconscious, and this was important both for him and for you. However, it meant rushing home after work, a quick meal, perhaps getting children into bed and finding a baby sitter, and again rushing to the hospital. It was a pace that no one could keep up for long, but you thought it would all be different when he was home again. Now the time has come for him to leave hospital, you realize that it may not be as simple as you thought, you wonder if it is right for him, and whether or not you will be able to cope. First, we need to look at the reasons for the move from hospital and how it works, and secondly, at possible alternatives.

WHY IS IT TIME TO LEAVE HOSPITAL?

You saw in Chapter 3 how Michael progressed from the Intensive Care Department to the Head-Injury Ward while he was in hospital. This happened when there was no longer any need for the life-support machinery, although he still needed to have expert nursing care for the whole 24-hour day. As he improved he was able to do more and more for himself, and at last he reached the stage where all his ordinary needs were a roof over his head, food, and a little help with the difficult things. Not only were the services of an acute hospital ward not needed any longer, but the atmosphere of sickness and bustle was bad for him. He was ready to move on.

WHERE TO GO: HOME OR SOMEWHERE ELSE?

As well as the basics of living, the head-injured victim has two other needs. One is to go back to living in the real world, supported by family and friends, and with the sense of security that this brings. Parents will want to provide this support, because this is what they have done over the years when their children were growing up, through the trials of chicken pox and mumps, broken bones, school reports, and adolescence. Wives will want to look after the husbands that they love, and vice versa. Friends will want to show that nothing has changed.

Going back home must be the first choice. It is the nearest thing to normal, the surroundings are familiar, and the patient will be among family. Sometimes, of course, this is not possible because of circumstances; there may not be room, a parent or spouse may be sick, or there may be some other barrier.

Although home may be the obvious choice, in some circumstances it is not always the best choice. Indeed there can be real disadvantages. The first is that a person who has had a head injury can be very difficult to deal with. Often he is not aware of his own behaviour, and he loses the consideration for others which makes family life possible. He is often irritable and sensitive to noise made by other people. He may want to do unsuitable or unsafe things, like playing the stereo at midnight, or insisting on taking his motorbike out for a spin. (You will read about these problems in the next chapter.) In many cases he has been used to living his own life, making his own decisions, and it can be very difficult for family to exert enough authority and firmness to control this sort of situation. The shift from the role of loving parent or spouse to that of a firm guardian is a very difficult one to make, and a situation can develop that is destructive both to the family and the head-injured person.

In-hospital needs	After-hospital needs
Life support	Food and shelter
Intensive care	Supervision
24-hour nursing	Family and friends
	Rehabilitation

We have already said that there are two needs, one being to return to living in the everyday world. The other is for formal rehabilitation treatment, the treatment which will get movement and balance back to normal, which will get the victim to think properly, and to return to the occupation and skills which he had before the accident. Some of this can be achieved by a home programme arranged by the hospital therapists but much of it needs to be done under expert supervision. This means frequent visits to the hospital or rehabilitation centre. If it is a long way away, there may be problems with transport, and the travelling may cause so much tiredness that the treatment does less good. If this is the case then it may be best to live in at a rehabilitation centre. Going home for weekends can then become a real holiday and enjoyed by everyone.

In ideal circumstances, the pros and cons of leaving hospital and going either home or to a residential rehabilitation centre would be worked out on the facts of each case, and a trial made of what seemed to be the better choice, always with the chance of changing if it seemed good to do so. It is unfortunate that this rational choice is often not possible. There may be no centre, or a waiting list which is often so long that there is a destructive gap between application and acceptance. Out-patient rehabilitation may be all that is available.

People with less severe head injuries

Many people will stay in the Head-Injury Ward for only a few days and they will recover to the extent that home is the obvious place to go. This does not mean that some of the problems that we have described above will not occur. A person who seems to have made a very good recovery in the controlled surroundings of a hospital ward may still become irritable when he has to deal with noisy children or neighbours, and he may not accept that he is neither fit to drive, nor well enough to go to the pub for a drink. In most cases this stage lasts for a short time only, and provided that you have been warned about the problems and advised how to cope, (see Chapter 5) you should get by without too much trouble.

Many hospitals have a system where the patient is given an appointment to come back to see the doctor in two or three weeks' time. At this stage usually some tests will be done to check the person's ability to concentrate, and to check how well memory and reaction times have recovered. This is the stage where the decision will be made about whether he should begin the return to work or school, or be started on a rehabilitation programme.

A person with a less severe head injury, who has not been admitted to hospital, usually misses out on this care. Because of the numbers involved, it would be very expensive to include every patient in the system outlined in the last paragraph. However, it should be possible to provide a service for the 5–10 per cent of patients from this group who will need continuing care. (One such service is described in Chapter 7.)

People who are not well enough to go home

Some people with very severe head-injuries make little progress after they leave intensive care. They move and speak very little, they do not respond very much to what is going on around them, and they remain dependent on others even for basic needs such as feeding and toileting. Their care in the Head-Injury Ward, where people are expected to be progressing, becomes inappropriate, and the hospital needs to move them somewhere else.

Only very rarely, perhaps in the case of young children, is it possible for the patient to go home, because of the burden of their care. Some health districts have special accommodation for the patient, but in many cases publicly funded or private geriatric hospitals are the only possibilities. These may (sometimes they do not) provide a level of care that is adequate to keep the victim alive and free from complications. However, it is rare for them to continue with a programme based on the expectation of further improvement. It is a fact, however, that if a patient does receive continued rehabilitation then he can continue to improve, although very slowly, and he sometimes may achieve sufficient recovery to make the difference between total dependence and at least partial self care.

HOW IS LEAVING THE HOSPITAL ORGANIZED?

When the transfer is to a nursing home, or if you are lucky to a rehabilitation facility, the date and time the patient leaves the acute hospital is set to suit both places. But you as the parent or family member are entitled to be kept fully informed of the arrangements. Even though the transfer is to another medical facility, you should make sure that you work through the rest of this chapter, which suggests the things that should be done before a patient leaves the hospital which he has been in since the accident.

If you are going to look after your friend or relative at home, there need to be arrangements which will make sure that you will be able to cope before he is handed over to your care. A system which works well, and which is followed by many acute-care hospitals, has three stages. The time of each stage should be set by a meeting of family members, medical and nursing staff, rehabilitation therapists, and usually the social worker assigned to your case. The patient may also be present if he is able to take part in the discussion. Before the first meeting or 'case conference', the occupational therapist may have visited your home to see what modifications will be needed to make it practical for the victim to live with you. If he will still be in a wheelchair when he goes home, for example, then access to the house must be looked at and modifications made so that he can use the bathroom and the toilet.

The first home-stay stage is usually a day visit. You might pick the victim up in your car, or ambulance transport might be arranged to bring him home and later return him to the hospital. If you manage this without too many problems, then the victim can have weekend leave, where he stays at home overnight on a Saturday evening. Again, after discussion of any problems, and after modifications have been made to overcome these problems, you move on to the final stage, which is full discharge home from hospital.

The three stages to leaving hospital
Day visit
Weekend leave
Discharge

Before he leaves the hospital, make an appointment to see the doctor who is in charge of your friend or relative. Make a list of the things you want to know about. Remember that this specialist is a busy person who is likely to have unscheduled emergencies which interrupt your visit with him, so allow enough time before the date set for discharge to fit in another appointment if necessary.

You will want to ask the specialist about the medication which the patient may be taking, and who you should go to to renew the prescription, or to make a decision about when it can be stopped. You will also want to ask about a follow-up appointment for him to be seen by the doctor in charge, or by a member of the team. If the victim is going to a rehabilitation centre, find out how you can get to see and talk to whoever will be looking after them there.

If you will be looking after your relative or friend at home, you will need to check that arrangements have been made for him to have any out-patient treatment which may be needed, and that you know the name and contact phone number for the person who has overall responsibility for his rehabilitation.

Many areas have support groups for families and care-givers where you can talk with other people who have had the same experiences as you. If you have not already done so, make sure that you make contact with your local group before the patient leaves hospital. This is the time when you will need all the support that you can get. It is also important to make sure that arrangements are made before the patient comes home from hospital for the practical help which you might need. In some countries, for example, if he still has difficulty with bladder control then you can get bedding and sleepwear provided and laundered by the extramural hospital. Ask your social worker about what help may be available in your case.

The time that the victim is in hospital is the time when you should have most direct access to rehabilitation officers and to social workers. Make sure that these people understand your family circumstances. This is the time to find out what financial help you are entitled to. For example, if you will need to take time off work to look after your friend or family member some accident insurance schemes allow for you to be reimbursed for loss of wages. Your social worker will be able to tell you about other allowances. Do not be too proud to take advantage of these. Money will not compensate you for the effects of the accident, but it may make the difference between being able to afford labour-saving help and struggling to balance the budget on a reduced income, with the extra expense that is entailed in caring for a head-injured victim.

If the friend or relative that you will be looking after at home is still not able to walk, make sure that you have been shown how to get him and the wheelchair into your car. If you do not have your own transport, check that arrangements have been made by the hospital to bring him back for out-patient appointments. Check also about how this is to be paid for. The expense of even a short journey can become a burden if this journey has to be repeated five or six days a week for months on end. Again, check with your social worker or rehabilitation officer to see if you can get reimbursed for this.

Before you take the patient home from hospital

have you:

asked about medication?

asked about out-patient treatment?

been given the name of your contact person?

contacted a family support group?

found out about financial help?

found out about practical help?

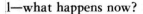

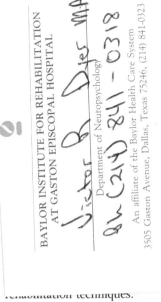

s a magic word. If only their relative or
on centre, or have physiotherapy every
n their problems would all be fixed. It is
ie a shortfall in rehabilitation resources
 the condition. This is not to say that
ut it is equally important to be aware of
natic brain damage means.
l in an accident they do not grow again.
ems, because most of us have millions
se, and one of the theories about why
brain injury is that new brain pathways
re' cells. These new pathways will be
tinuously practises the actions that have
and more repetition is the basis of most
rehabilitation techniques.

The rehabilitation team

Depending on the injuries of your friend or family member he will work
with some or all of the following rehabilitation team members:

Physiotherapists (physical therapists)

The physiotherapist aims to help patients recover the ability to use the
muscles in their arms, legs, neck, and trunk, so that they can sit and
stand without losing their balance, and co-ordinate their movements.
Exercises may range from practice in leg movements, so that they can
walk again, to practice in fine hand movements, so that they can use
a pen.

Occupational therapists

The occupational therapist aims to help patients carry out everyday
tasks. Exercises can range from showing them how to dress themselves
and to carry out their own toilet, to teaching them about budgeting and
managing their own finances. The occupational therapist will also
provide special equipment to help them to be as independent as possible,
even though they may have considerable physical handicaps.

Speech therapists

The speech and language therapist aims to help patients communicate with other people, using both spoken and written words. This means that they could have exercises in reading and writing, as well as exercises aimed at giving them practice in understanding what people are saying to them. The speech therapist may also give them practice in remembering what they have read and heard.

Neuropsychologists

The neuropsychologist has a special interest in cognitive skills; those skills such as memory, perception, and understanding that are needed for us to gain knowledge. He or she aims to find what abilities the patient has, what skills have been affected by the injury, and in what way. If there is a memory problem, for example, is this just a problem when words have to be remembered, is the problem mainly in getting things into memory, or in getting things out again at some later stage? The aim is to find out what areas need exercise. The neuropsychologist will see the patients regularly during rehabilitation, to make sure that the cognitive re-training exercises that they have been doing are helping them to regain the skills that they have lost.

Cognitive retraining therapists

In some centres cognitive retraining is carried out by the neuropsychologist, in some by the occupational therapist, and in other centres the speech therapist does this. In each case the aim is to teach the patient to regain the skills that have been lost or impaired. Sometimes this is done by teaching them to use the skills that have not been affected by the accident to help them carry out activities that are hard for them because of the brain injury.

Social workers

Social workers are skilled in helping families get the practical help that is needed. They know which community and government facilities are available, and they will often be involved in finding somewhere for the patient to go when it is time to leave hospital. Social workers are also often involved in running support groups, either for the victims themselves or for the families.

Clinical psychologists

The clinical psychologist is a skilled counsellor, and will help you all cope with the changes that the accident has brought about. He or she will also be able to help if the victim's behaviour is causing management problems.

Rehabilitation officers

Some accident insurance schemes employ rehabilitation officers who will act as co-ordinators of different services. Their involvement will sometimes continue until the victim has either made a full recovery, or until the recovery has 'plateaued', until there has been no improvement over several months.

The rehabilitation team

Physiotherapist (physical therapist)
Occupational therapist
Speech therapist
Neuropsychologist
Cognitive retraining therapist
Social worker
Clinical psychologist
Rehabilitation officer

What can you expect from rehabilitation?

Rehabilitation aims to help people who have had head injuries reach their potential level of recovery. At one end of the scale are victims who eventually will be able to do all the activities which they did before their accidents at a similar level of skill. At the other end of the scale there will be victims who may be able to do nothing except breathe for themselves, even years after the injury. For these people, extensive expenditure of rehabilitation time and effort is needed to make any difference to how they do, and their potential for recovery is limited.

In most cases there is the problem that 'potential recovery' is something that is difficult to measure. We can of course keep a record of 'partial recovery', how much recovery people have made at fixed periods of time after the injury. Does failure to find any improvement from one period to the next mean that the patients have reached their potential? Is this as well as they are likely to get? Not necessarily. It does suggest, however, that the patients have reached the stage when the effort that is being spent on their rehabilitation is not accompanied by equivalent returns.

At this point the rehabilitation team will probably suggest that the treatment is cut back, or they may give the victim a three or six month break from treatment. They may explain to you that they need to concentrate their efforts on patients who will get more benefit from the time which they spend with them. This is often a difficult decision for families to accept. It is important to remember that the pattern of recovery after neurological damage is usually one of rapid gains early after injury, and much slower gains, even pauses, in recovery after that. For this reason, the break in treatment is not necessarily the end of rehabilitation for your friend or family member. It is important that you make sure that you have been given a definite appointment time when progress can be checked, and when the decision to reduce treatment can be reviewed.

Rehabilitation—magic cures

It is often at the stage when recovery seems to have stopped that the search for a magic cure begins. There is the belief that somehow, somewhere, there will be rehabilitation for the victim's head injury that will fix things. Usually this magic cure is in another country or state. Often it is something that you have read about in the popular press. It usually involves considerable expense because it is not recognized as part of orthodox rehabilitation medicine, and so it is not covered by your accident insurance. Often it involves considerable sacrifices of personal and family life, because you and your family have to be the practitioners of this therapy. One of the inevitable consequences of this is that you are then responsible for the success or failure of the treatment. It is inevitable that families feel some guilt about the circumstances of the accident, no matter how tenuous the cause for blame. It is tragic when another source of guilt is added if the magic does not work.

Of course, just because a treatment is unorthodox or costly or time-consuming does not necessarily make it useless or ineffective. However, it does not necessarily mean that it does work. Before you commit yourself to any new course of action, first of all talk it over with the co-ordinator of the rehabilitation programme. Find out what the magic cure offers that the conventional programme does not. It may be possible to try out new exercises at home using rehabilitation staff the victim is familiar with, without the effort and expense of travelling miles to a strange place. Sometimes the only difference is in the quantity of treatment, and more is not necessarily better for the head-injured patient. Remember that one of his main problems is that he tires very quickly, and when the brain is tired the only thing that extra exercise will do is to tire him even further.

It is also helpful to discuss the decision to try out the new treatment with your family doctor, who should be able to warn you if it may prove harmful in your case. You need also to bring it up with your family support group, so that you can find out if there are other families who have tried the magic cure. Finally, never commit yourself to a programme or centre on the spur of the moment. Wait till you have all the information that you can get, and take all the advice that you can, particularly advice from people who do not have anything to gain from your decision, or who do not have a special interest in the proposed treatment.

Rehabilitation in isolated country areas

We have talked about the lack of appropriate rehabilitation centres, and pointed out that this is a problem which is universal. The problem is even greater if you live in an area away from a main centre, as even the most ambitious and wealthy health system cannot be expected to provide facilities in every town and village in the country. What do you do if you live in a geographically isolated area?

The first decision that you will be faced with is, should you move to a bigger centre where your friend or relative can get the help that is needed? Obviously this will depend on your family circumstances, but in general you should not be hasty about doing this. Certainly you need to discuss the feasibility of the move with all the members of your family. The head-injured member is not the only one who needs to be considered. You also need to discuss alternative plans with your social worker. It may be possible to find residential accommodation for the victim, or for him to be given a rehabilitation programme that he can do at home.

If you follow a rehabilitation programme at home then your first need will be for information and advice. One of the reasons for writing this book was to cater for people who do not have access to face-to-face counselling about head injury. But since no book can be a substitute for interaction with other people, it is important that you arrange for some sort of personal contact. This may be with a staff member at the hospital where your relative or friend was nursed immediately after the accident. It is also important that you attend at least one support group meeting before taking the patient home, so that you can set up a network of people you can write to when you need to get things off your chest. Finally, it is especially important to make sure that the social worker finds out about what extra help you may be entitled to as a resident in an isolated area.

CASE HISTORIES

Michael

Michael's mother and father were delighted when they were given the news that Michael was well enough to go home from hospital. His father accepted that it was best for Michael to stay with his mother, and Michael himself agreed to this, seeing it as a temporary measure until he returned to his university studies and his own flat.

The first weeks went reasonably smoothly. Michael spent a large part of the day asleep, and his mother was able to use these periods to catch up on housework and organize meals. This was because while Michael was awake he was very demanding. He became upset if his mother did not stay in the same room as him, and he followed her wherever she went. He was very forgetful, and he became quite angry whenever he could not find what he needed. He did not seem to enjoy reading as he used to, and his mother learned that he was happiest when she played cards or chess with him.

Friends and relatives visited often at first to help keep him amused. Some were better than others at knowing how to handle him, and at knowing when Michael had had enough. His father was not particularly good at coping with Michael. He was embarrassed and upset when Michael lost his temper, he found it hard to accept that Michael's memory was poor, and that he sometimes did childish things. The time between visits became longer and longer, until eventually he stopped coming. His way of coping with Michael at this stage was to not have to see him and the changes that the accident had brought.

Mary

Mary's first words, three days after her accident, were that she wanted to go home. Every day the departure of her parents from the ward initiated a flood of tears and a flood of heart-rending pleas ('Don't leave me mummy', 'daddy, *please* take me home, please, please', and so on). This placed considerable stress on the hospital staff, as well as on her parents, and Mary was sent home for weekend leave as soon as she was considered medically stable. This weekend leave turned out to be complete discharge, because Mary made such a scene on Sunday evening when she was to go back to the hospital that her mother eventually gave in. So Mary became an out-patient, at a time when she still occasionally wet her bed, when she still occasionally choked on her food, and when she still, most of the time, asked the same questions over and over again, because her memory had not yet started to work properly.

Mary's mum, a registered nurse, applied for and was granted the three months leave that she had accumulated. The family coped reasonably well for this three months. Mary's mother was able to get the other members of the family organized and off to work and school before Mary woke. Then, with just the two of them, she had plenty of time to rouse Mary, to get her bathed and dressed and fed, and to take her to the hospital for her twice-weekly paediatric out-patient sessions.

She also had time, before the other children returned from school, to 'teach' Mary herself. She was pleased that Mary played her favourite game (Monopoly) with as much skill as she had before her accident. She was a little uneasy about Mary's reluctance to do jigsaw puzzles, which had also been a favourite pastime. She was also bothered by Mary's complete lack of enthusiasm about gifts of the colouring and perceptual puzzle books that had formerly been her favourite sort of present. Partly because of these worries, Mary's mother turned more and more to purely physical activities, and she was able to make out a good case to herself that Mary needed exercise, and walking, swimming, and horse-riding were good rehabilitation for her.

Three months went by very quickly, and Mary's mother was faced with the decision about returning to work, and what would happen to Mary. She sought help in making this decision from the appropriate agencies, because she knew the system. However, even though she had this advantage, she was still left with the decision of whether she would devote all her time to looking after Mary, or whether she would continue with her career. She chose the latter, using the very sound and solid reasons that her salary was needed to cover the mortgage on the family home, and that she needed to consider all her children, not just Mary.

A family meeting was held with the members of the rehabilitation team to plan how Mary's care could be shared once her mother went back to work. Mary's father did not attend this meeting. He still found it very difficult to accept the way the accident had changed his favourite daughter, and his method of coping was to ignore the whole incident. However, the meeting went ahead without him. It was decided to increase the time Mary spent at the rehabilitation centre to a full five day week. The social worker arranged for an attendant to care for her for an hour each afternoon until her parents returned from work. Mary's mother had arranged to work a permanent day shift, to coincide with the time Mary was at the centre. It was an optimistic meeting, and even Mary was pleased with the plans, and not unhappy about losing her mother's undivided attention.

Unfortunately, the plans did not work as well in practice. Mary became very tired with a full week programme, and even though her therapist allowed her two sleep periods during the day instead of the usual one, by Friday she was exhausted and hard to cope with. The attendant care scheme worked well at the beginning, but when a new attendant had to be found because the original lady moved out of the area, the social worker had difficulty finding a suitable replacement. The eventual choice was a person who was not as sympathetic to Mary's needs as she should have been, and there was continual friction between her and Mary. Finally, Mary's mother discovered that her own ability to cope with her family was reduced as she had fewer hours to spend with them, and less energy at the end of her working day.

Arnold

As soon as Arnold regained consciousness the day after the accident, he began to worry about his business affairs, and the need to get out of hospital. Because he was obviously still a little confused, and also quite unsteady on his feet, his doctors were not happy about him going home to an empty house. Eventually his 21-year-old daughter arranged to take a week off work so that she could be home with him. While she was there Arnold managed well. She made the phone calls that he wanted made, organized a temporary manager for the restaurant, and watched that her father was not over-tiring himself.

Arnold's problems started when his daughter's week was up. He had been convinced that he could manage on his own, because he had felt relaxed and stress free with his daughter there to keep the pressure off him. He managed badly on his own. He forgot important phone calls, or he made phone calls and forgot why he had made them. He insisted on checking the restaurant books, he became muddled and confused, and he became so irritable and aggressive that his chef threatened to walk out. His lady friend called to take him for a meal and became distressed when she found that he had completely forgotten their date. This upset Arnold, who uncharacteristically burst into tears.

So it went on. Arnold did not need to be in hospital, but it was obvious that he was not coping with being at home. He was too proud to ask his daughter to return for another few weeks, and too uncomfortable about his relationship with his friend to accept her offer for him to stay with her.

5. The continuing effects of head injury

When the staff at the hospital talked to you about what the future might hold for your relative or friend, they probably used the terms 'brain damage' or 'brain injury'. Obviously the outcome depends on the amount of damage, but the words suggest a gloomy outlook to most people. The amount of recovery that you have seen up until the time the head-injured person is ready to leave hospital will have been a great source of reassurance to you, and you are right to assume that it will continue. You need to realize, however, that although the victim is well enough to leave hospital, there are many problems still to be faced. If you know about these in advance then you will be better prepared to deal with them.

In this chapter we describe the problems ahead, and explain why they occur. We also give you some suggestions about how to cope with them. These are problems which almost every person who has had a head injury will experience, although each will have an individual mixture. In Chapter 6 we will describe the special problems which only a proportion of people will experience.

FATIGUE

Without doubt, fatigue is one of the most limiting after-effects of head injury, because it influences everything that is done. The victim will find that after every activity he will tire much more quickly than he expects, whether he is trying to concentrate, take exercise, or just talk socially. Even activities which are normally relaxing, like watching television, will tire him. Why this should be is not yet known, but it seems likely that the injury has damaged the part of the brain which controls the rhythm of sleeping and waking. This is not surprising, as the first effect of a head injury is coma, a very deep sort of sleep.

Someone who is fit and well wakes in the morning feeling fresh. The well person can work right through the day until he starts to feel tired, a word we use to describe the feeling that everything needs much more effort. If a person goes on working when he is tired he gets careless, and the quality of the work deteriorates. At last it becomes too unpleasant, there are too many mistakes however hard he tries, and he has to stop.

After a good night's rest he is fresh again and can go back to work. It looks as if he starts the day with a measured amount of energy, he can work until this is exhausted, when this happens he becomes tired and inefficient, and then he can get the energy back by a good night's sleep.

A head-injured person can feel fresh when he wakes, but within a short time, an hour or two or maybe less, the feeling of tiredness comes on and, much more quickly than the well person, his performance deteriorates and he has to stop. When he takes a rest or sleep it does him less good than he expects. Even if he gets a good night's sleep, he may not feel fresh the next morning. What seems to be happening is that he starts with much less energy, uses it up more quickly, and has difficulty in getting it back by resting. The next day he is still in 'energy-debt' so that the symptoms start even sooner.

There are other disturbances of the sleeping and waking mechanism. After head injury more time may be spent in the lighter stages of sleep, which are less refreshing. As a result of this the quality of dreaming may change, sometimes with nightmares, and sometimes with very little dreaming at all.

> If your head-injured friend says that he is too tired to go out with you, he probably is.

It is often very difficult for a person who has had a head injury to understand the needs of this situation. We are all brought up to believe that we can 'do better if we try harder' and the reaction to fatigue is often dogged perseverance and a determination to finish the job. This usually results in a downward spiral of deterioration.

Families and rehabilitation staff need to act as monitors of the head-injured person's energy use, to make sure that he stays within the limits where he will be able to function effectively. The rehabilitation team will organize the treatment times so that periods which are 'energy-draining' are alternated with periods of rest, when his batteries can be recharged. Families will monitor the home and leisure activities to make sure that he is not overdoing things. To do this, families need to appreciate that the signs that he is over-tired are not necessarily that he will want to lie down or sit in a chair. Indeed, often the opposite is true. He can become more restless, more distractable, more disorganized, or more talkative. His mood may seem exaggerated, he may be quicker to laugh or to argue and less easy to reason with, or he may withdraw and refuse to discuss anything; yet he may deny that he is tired, even though this is very obvious to you.

It will be difficult to persuade him to do the only sensible thing, that is, to take some rest. This is why it is important that the care-givers monitor the amount of activity, and are able to direct the head-injured person to rest before he gets to the 'over-tired' stage. Often there are very clear signals that your relative or friend has exceeded the energy level and is approaching this overload. You need to watch out for these signals. Some of the most frequent are unusual pallor, a drawn tense look, or a rather glazed expression in the eyes.

If you can recognize the early signs of fatigue in your relative or friend, you can help him by directing him to stop or change what he is doing, and to husband his energies. This should be the first priority in managing the problem. The second priority is to protect him from well-meaning associates who do not understand the basis of his tiredness. As an example, if you know that he does not have the energy to watch a video (which involves concentrating on the screen, remembering the plot, the characters, what they said, and so on) you can dissuade his associates from pressuring him to join them. The third priority of fatigue management is that of communication. You need to keep the rehabilitation team informed of any unusually tiring activity that your relative or friend has taken up, or anything different that he has done which has made him more tired than normal, or importantly, has affected his ability to cope with rehabilitation.

Unfortunately, even when the early obvious fatigue effects are past the head-injured person will still need to manage his energy level carefully. He will need to plan to have extra rest periods if he has an unusual or demanding activity coming up. He will also need to be aware that it may take two or three days for him to recover from this activity.

Managing fatigue

Monitor activities
Ensure frequent rest periods, especially after tiring
   activities
Protect from well-meaning friends
Communicate with rehabilitation staff

POOR CONCENTRATION AND ATTENTION

Problems with concentration are closely linked to tiredness, and probably have the same basic cause. When we talk about impaired concentration there are three different ways in which this will affect what the head-injured person can do.

Focused attention

The first is that he will find it hard to keep his attention focused on one thing. He will find it hard to concentrate on doing a rehabilitation exercise, for example, and ignore what is going on in the room around him. You will find that when you talk to him he is easily distracted and cannot ignore trivial movements or noises. Anything is likely to grab his attention, even things that you have not noticed. This is because we are normally able to use part of our attention mechanism to keep track of what is going on around us, while we focus our attention on what we are doing. The head-injured person is unable to do this. For this reason the rehabilitation staff will usually try to treat him in a quiet room on his own, to reduce the number of things that might distract him. It is important that you also watch out for this. As an example, if he still needs to put all his attention into keeping his balance when he walks, talking to him at the same time is not the right thing to do!

Divided attention

The second, related, way in which the problem which the head-injured person has with concentrating will show is when he tries to divide his attention between two things at the same time. Normally we do this without thinking about it. For example, whenever we write down a telephone message, take notes during a lecture, or look after a child while listening to a friend talk, we are using this special skill. After a head injury the victim does not have enough concentration to focus on one task, so it is not surprising that he cannot cope with two. The best way to help him through this stage is to arrange things so that he does not have to divide his attention between several sources. Try to restrict visitors to one at a time, for example.

Attention span

The third way in which poor attention is shown is in the length of time that the head-injured person is able to concentrate on a task—the concentration span. In the early stages this can be as short as five minutes. The rehabilitation staff will take this into account, knowing that there is no point in expecting him to stick at an exercise once he has exhausted his ability to concentrate. Family and friends need to understand too that he may be capable of doing something at one point in time, then be unable to continue a short time later. The family should keep in mind how long the 'attention span' is, and not expect him to concentrate for longer than this. It is reassuring to know that the concentration span will get longer as the weeks go by. It is also important to remember that when a head-injured person is tired his concentration will be even worse. You can encourage him to plan his days so that the toughest tasks are tackled while he is fresh and alert. He also needs to be reassured that the right thing to do is to take rests, or have a sleep if he feels tired, rather than to try to finish what he is doing in one sitting and probably fail at it.

Problems of concentration

Difficulties with:
focused attention—ignoring distraction
divided attention—e.g. taking lecture notes
attention span—how long does concentration last?

MEMORY PROBLEMS

It will be easier to understand how memory can go wrong after a head injury if you know the way that memory normally works. It is important to realize that it is not a simple one-stage system. There are several steps that have to be carried through. Before we can remember something we first have to notice it, or attend to it. Next we have to store it in the brain, and it has to be stored in such a way that we can get it back later when we want to recall it. It then has to stay safe in storage, and lastly to be able to be recalled when it is needed.

The next fact about 'normal' memory is that there are differences in the way memories are stored, depending on whether or not they contain information that we will try to get back to later. Not all of the things we have to remember every day have to be remembered for very long. A telephone number can be remembered for as long as it takes to make a call, but it may never be used again and so it can be forgotten safely. Other things we may never forget as long as we live. This tells us that some memories are permanent and others only temporary. Things we have known for a long time, a childhood memory or the words of our native language, are permanent memories which are unlikely to be lost, and which seem to be stored in a different way in the brain to new information. Things that we have known for a short time only, such as the name of a new acquaintance, or a new phone number, are more easily forgotten. However, some temporary memories can later become permanent if conditions are right. This happens when we have a use for that memory and refer to it or recall it frequently. This regular use or exercise of a memory makes it more likely to endure and eventually become a permanent memory. We all make use of this fact when we study. We know that if we rehearse something often enough we will be able to remember it when we need to. Of course, the opposite is also true. If we make no use of newly learned information we will quickly forget it.

There is one other fact about how memory works which we need to understand in order to understand how a head injury can affect it. This is the concept of separate memory 'factories'. Memories of conversations, pictures, maps, or smells appear to be handled separately by the brain. For example, different parts of the brain work together to remember faces than are used to remember the names that go with those faces. In the same way, different parts of the brain are used to remember maps or diagrams than are used to remember a poem.

Stages of memory

Attend

Store (different stores for different memories):

(a) for short time (temporary memory)

(b) for later recall (long-term memory)

Remember:

(a) without any hints (recall)

(b) when a clue is given (recognition)

Memory is thus a very complex system, and there are many different stages and parts of this system which can be affected by head injury. It is also usual for some parts of the system to work perfectly well, which often makes it hard for friends and relatives to understand why their head-injured victim can be said to have a 'memory problem'. Most patients have no trouble recalling permanent memories which were laid down before the accident, but many have difficulty laying down new memories in some or all of the memory 'factories'. Thus your relative or friend may be able to recall details of a family gathering that happened years ago and that you had almost forgotten. You will understand now, we hope, that this does not mean that he or she has a good memory, but simply that the ability to recall permanent memories has not been affected.

We have not yet discussed the memory problem that head-injured persons are most likely to be concerned about. This is the memory gap around the accident. The head-injured person cannot remember what happened to him, or how it happened. Sometimes he will have no memory of things that happened for a while before the injury. He will also have another sort of memory loss for things that happened after the injury. Not only can he not remember the time that he was unconscious, but he cannot remember some of the time after he woke up, even though he may have spent this time apparently awake and talking with friends and family. These two sorts of memory loss are sometimes called retrograde amnesia and post-traumatic amnesia.

Retrograde amnesia

At the moment of injury the brain stops noticing and storing memories. This is why there is rarely any memory of the injury itself, although occasionally things happening up to the instant itself may be remembered. More usually, the last clear memory of the head-injured person may be of something that happened some minutes, hours, days, months, or even years before. Sometimes the victim will remember a few things that fall within this time of otherwise total memory loss. Usually these memories are of special significance, such as a family wedding.

As he gets better he may remember a few more of the things that happened before the injury, but he is unlikely to remember everything. In particular he is unlikely to remember the instant of the injury itself. This is why it is pointless for him to waste energy trying to remember it, and why you do not need to worry about the emotional effect it might have on him if he does get this memory back. He can never remember the accident, because he does not have that memory in his brain. The moment of impact interrupted the mechanism where the brain changes things that are experienced into a form which makes it possible for them to be remembered later. The things that happened immediately before and at the time of the impact did not have time to be changed into memories, so they can never be remembered.

Post-traumatic amnesia

Even after a fairly minor head injury there will be a time after the head-injured person has apparently 'woken up' which he will later be unable to remember. This time can range from a few seconds or minutes to days, weeks, or months. During this period he may answer or ask questions, he may walk around, have a meal, or do other apparently 'awake' things, but because he is completely unable to remember them later we know that he was obviously not actually awake. It may help to understand this stage if you compare it to sleepwalking. We are not usually surprised that we do not remember things that happen while we are asleep. In the same way, do not expect your relative or friend to remember what happened during this stage. He has not woken up enough to have the ability to put things which happen into memory store.

Earlier we explained how it is unreasonable to expect a head-injured person to have a good memory if he is not able to attend to what goes on around him. Because problems with concentration and attention are so very common in the early days after the injury, memory problems are also very common at that time, and often improved concentration is accompanied by improved memory. When this does not happen, it suggests that the breakdown is because he has problems storing memories in the brain, or maybe problems in getting stored memories out again when he needs them.

Coping with a poor memory

The first step in dealing with a memory problem is to find out where the problem is. For this reason your relative or friend will have seen a neuro-psychologist, and you and the rehabilitation staff will know which parts of the system he can manage, and which parts have been affected by the injury. Memory re-training will make use of this information. If the problem is in putting things into memory store, for example, a head-injured person will be taught ways of doing this more effectively. The same applies to problems with retrieval, that is, of getting something out of memory when you want to. Or it may be that the 'memory factory' that handles words is still able to work, but the one that deals with pictures is rather useless. In these cases, exercises will concentrate on teaching him how to use the good 'word factory' to remember pictures, by translating the important parts of these pictures into words.

However, any kind of memory retraining is very labour-intensive, and there is no guarantee that it will work. In contrast, the technique of making memory 'external' gives immediate success. Making memory external simply means that pressure is taken off the brain by writing down things that have to be remembered. By using notepads, by making lists, by using calendars and diaries, a head-injured person can increase greatly the capacity of his memory. The rehabilitation team can give advice on the ways that will work best for individual cases. In situations where it is very important that nothing is forgotten, for example, a pocket tape recorder may be more useful than trying to take notes. It will never be possible to make faulty memory into fault-free memory, but by limiting the number of things that the head-injured person forgets he can regain a degree of control over his life. He is now in charge of the memory problem rather than the other way around.

> **Writing things down is an excellent way of coping with a poor memory. It does not hinder recovery.**

You as the care-giver can help him to establish a routine to make sure that looking in the diary, or checking the calendar, become part of daily life. You can also help by reassuring him that managing the memory problem in this way, by taking much of the load off internal memory, is the most effective way of helping that memory to work.

LACK OF INSIGHT

Insight is knowing how well you are able to do things. When your head-injured friend or family member lacks insight he cannot appreciate the way in which other people react to what he does, and because of this he does not see the need to alter how he acts. This ability to judge the effect of what we say and do on other people, and to use this knowledge to modify our behaviour, is controlled by the front parts of the brain, behind the forehead. When this part of the brain is not working efficiently the person may genuinely believe that there is nothing wrong with him, or he may focus on a minor consequence of the accident, such as a stiff knee, and deny that he has any other problems. Of course, as long as he does not see that there is any need for it he will be unlikely to make much progress in rehabilitation. It will be hard to convince him that he should work at overcoming a concentration problem, for example, if he is sure that his concentration is as good as it ever was.

Not only does lack of insight make it hard for the rehabilitation staff, but it is also hard for families and care-givers. Because he is unable to appreciate the consequences of what he does, his behaviour may be impulsive and often potentially dangerous. For instance he may insist on driving a car or riding a motor cycle, even though the rehabilitation team may have forbidden this because his reaction times are too slow for him to be safe. Try to avoid this kind of situation from developing by removing the motor cycle, for example, or by anticipating when he might want to go out and offering to drive him. Lack of insight is most common in the early days after a severe head-injury, and in most cases the victim will also find it hard to concentrate and will have a poor memory. Because of this, it is usually possible to distract him if he attempts to do something where he or others may be harmed. However, you will need to be quite vigilant, and you should also make sure that you have reliable helpers to take your place so that your relative or friend is not left alone if you need to go out.

If the victim's insight is poor

He may deny that there are problems
He may not see the need for rehabilitation
He may endanger others by his actions

The carer must be very vigilant
The carer must enlist 'minders' when they are out

Insight will improve as the head-injured person gets better, but this is unlikely to happen overnight. One day he might be quite realistic, and the next deny that he has any problems. You can help by making him aware of what he can and cannot do. Discuss the problems with the rehabilitation team, and support them in their efforts to promote realism.

SLOWED REACTIONS

Because the brain still does not have the normal amount of energy, the head-injured person will be unable to do things as quickly or as efficiently as he could before the accident. This happens with mental as well as physical activities. You will also find that he can take much longer to do even fairly simple automatic activities, such as eating or cleaning the teeth. He will usually be unaware that he has been so slow, because he is doing these tasks as fast as his slowed-down brain will allow. Do not fall into the trap of thinking that he is being deliberately obstructive, or trying to get you upset because you will be late for whatever appointment you have arranged for him. Make sure that you plan ahead, and arrange to start getting him ready several hours before the deadline.

When he has to carry out some complex activity, such as making a decision, he may work so slowly that he does not finish the task at all, because by the time he gets to considering the alternatives he has usually forgotten what they all are. You must make allowances for this. In the early stages after head injury the victim needs to be protected from the physical danger which can result from coping with dangerous machinery, or driving a motor vehicle while he still has slowed reactions. The second way you can help your head-injured relative or friend is to protect him from the need to cope with complex problems. The rehabilitation team will help you work out how you can break up these problems into smaller parts that are easier for the head-injured person to cope with.

HEADACHE

Headaches occur frequently after even quite mild injury. This book cannot replace the medical advice that you will seek if your friend or family member is bothered by headaches. They can have many causes, and your doctor will need to investigate these. However, one of the most common causes, particularly when headaches occur for the first time many months after injury, is stress or tension. Often the headaches show that the victim is trying to do too much, and disappear when the activity that has brought on the headache is stopped. In other cases they can be a sign that he is becoming anxious and concerned about himself, his job, or his family life. A stress management programme is often useful, and he will usually find that when he has mastered some relaxation techniques he will be able to reduce the intensity of the headache, if not eliminate it completely.

EMOTIONAL UPS AND DOWNS

In the early stages after injury, there can be one of two emotional 'reactions' which are seen regardless of what happens around the head-injured person. At one extreme he may appear to be very happy, unconcerned by his plight and never troubled by sadness, even when told news which normally would distress him. At the other extreme he may show no emotion at all. He may appear uncaring, unmoved, unloving, and untouchable, almost as though his feelings have been lost. This is because one of the consequences of head injury can be that the person expresses emotion differently, or reacts differently in emotional situations. The early stage, whether of extreme elation or complete loss of feeling, is usually replaced by a stage where emotions appear to be running wild. There may be swings of mood, perhaps from a real 'high' to a desperate 'low'. Emotions not normally part of the personality may make themselves more obvious.

Our familiar emotional reactions are built up through long experience. The brain makes sense of our emotional experience so that we react in the right way. While growing up we learn to recognize signs of fear, anger, and other emotions in our own body. These are things that we do not think about doing, they just happen automatically. We know for certain, without any hesitation, that we are angry, happy, sad, or elated. A head injury can alter this way of experiencing the world for the victim. This is why ordinary everyday experiences suddenly have the potential to unsettle him or make him feel uncomfortable. Crowds of people, the noise and bustle of the street, and the babble of noisy places may all be experienced as unpleasant or even frightening. Emotions may be experienced in a confusing way, so that he is unsure just what he is feeling. The ability to gauge the emotional reactions of others, to tell by their faces if they are happy or sad, can be impaired by the injury.

Very often the victim loses the ability to control emotional reactions such as tears or laughter. Sometimes this shows itself in not being able to stop one of these reactions once it has started, long after the emotion associated with it has been spent. Sometimes the tears or laughter are triggered by an inappropriate (or even no) emotion. He may be unable to control tears whenever he feels excited, even if this excitement is brought on by a favourite sports team scoring a goal, or any attempt at concentration may bring on uncontrollable laughter, no matter how serious he feels at the time. For some head-injured people tears and laughter seem to be severed from feelings, and occur for no apparent reason. These reactions can be embarrassing for family and friends as well as for the head-injured person. He will need reassurance from you that you understand this behaviour, and that you will explain to those around if he is unable to do this himself. It is also important to remember that, as with all the other effects of the accident, ability to control emotion will fluctuate with fatigue. Make sure that he is rested if he has to cope with a situation which could trigger tears or laughter.

Other emotional responses which can be affected by head injury are irritability and aggression. This behaviour is very common when the victim is first waking up, and the response may be to lash out with a fist at anyone in range. He may also be unable to express feelings in any way other than aggression. As an example, he may grasp onto your hand, which you know is because he wants you to stay with him, but then he either squeezes your hand so hard that it hurts, or else pinches your flesh, or attempts to twist your finger. This is as much out of conscious control as is the vocabulary that he may use at this time, which is often full of swear words. You need to realize that the aggression and bad language is not directed specifically at you. You need also to realize that this is not something that you can 'talk over' and settle when he is better, because this period is one which he will not be able to remember later on.

Even after he has recovered enough to remember things that happen to him from day to day, he may be easily irritated by rather trivial things, and aggression can still be a problem. If he is difficult at home, you may be hurt to learn from the rehabilitation team that his behaviour when he is with them is very good. He does not lose his temper, he does not shout and swear, and he does not throw things. There is a very simple explanation for this. Paradoxical as it may seem, he behaves badly in your company because he feels safe with you, and knows that you love him too. He does not feel this way with any of the people at the rehabilitation centre and he expends considerable energy controlling the aggression, because he knows that if he 'blows up' there he is likely to be asked to leave. He can relax once he gets home, and in a very real sense you are the safety valve. You need to talk about this problem with the team. Although the head-injured person will not be able to cope with a standard anger management course at this stage, the team may be able to help him, and they certainly will be able to teach you how to manage these moods. Obviously if you do not discuss this with the team then they can have no idea that anger is a problem. It may also help you to ride out this stage if you can accept that the behaviour of the head-injured person is not a personal attack on you, and that things will really get better as time goes on.

We need to describe one more emotional response which typically occurs rather late in the recovery cycle. It is quite natural for a head-injured person to become depressed as he gets better and gains more insight. With insight comes the realization of how many losses there have been; loss of individual freedom, loss of mobility, loss of skills, and perhaps mental, physical, and emotional losses. The depressed mood is therefore a realistic reaction to the many losses that he has experienced.

This mood of despondency may come and go over days, weeks, or months. The victim may express feelings of frustration, anger, or despair, and may talk of ending it all. If you are worried that he might do himself an injury, or worse, then talk to your own doctor or to someone from the rehabilitation team, and make sure that it is checked out to your satisfaction. Note, however, that an emotional reaction of this sort, which can be alarming to family members and friends, is a positive sign of recovery. You cannot feel blue about your problems without first knowing what they are. This recognition is vital to the success of continuing rehabilitation. You can help the head-injured person to understand that this depression is a positive sign that he is getting better: if left to himself, he may decide that he is getting worse as he feels so much worse. This would only exacerbate his already anxious and confused state, and he may worry about all the awful things that must be happening inside his head.

Understanding and accepting depression or anxiety as a natural and healthy reaction allows the rehabilitation to proceed in a positive way. Depression viewed this way is a step on the path to recovery.

Stages in emotional control

Early stage:
either over-happy or
no emotions

(cont.)

Stages in emotional control (cont.)

Middle stage:
over-reaction
irritability
aggression
inappropriate tears/laughter

Later stage:
ability to control moods with strangers
depressed
may still over-react

CHANGES IN SEXUALITY

The sexuality of the victim can be disturbed because of physical, psychological, or social changes. Impotence is a common problem, but one which the victim may feel unable or unwilling to talk about with the rehabilitation staff, or with his relatives or friends. In the early stages fatigue will be a causative factor, and so time may bring a solution. However, even in these early stages he should talk over the problem with a doctor, if you can persuade him to do this.

Psychological changes can arise because of the way head-injured people see themselves following the accident. Loss, scarring, or paralysis of limbs can seriously affect the self-image, leading to problems in dealing with social or sexual partners. Less obvious losses such as a change in job status can also lead to a loss of confidence in social situations, or a loss of self-esteem.

In social situations he may unwittingly break unwritten rules. For example, he may infringe on 'personal space' by moving too close when talking to someone, and nobody likes to feel pressured in this way. Neither are people likely to be impressed if the head-injured person forgot to clean his teeth or to take a shower. He may appear forward, touch people when he ought not to, or make jokes which are in bad taste. This type of behaviour can be seen as sexually provocative or out of place. Social rule breaking is common after a head injury, and it comes about because the victim no longer has the ability to judge the effect of the things he does on other people.

If your head-injured friend or relative behaves in a sexually inappropriate way, you can help him to change by pointing out why the things that he does are unacceptable. If possible, show him a way of doing things, or a way of expressing his feelings, which is socially acceptable. Do not expect quick results because the problem has its basis in impaired brain function. You may feel embarrassed and unable to talk about this behaviour with the head-injured person. In this case, discuss the problem with whichever member of the rehabilitation team you feel most comfortable with. He or she will understand, and will also be able to talk with the victim about your worries.

If you are caring for a head-injured person who lived independently before the accident then you have to allow him some independence in your new living arrangement. Too often parents fall into the trap of treating their adult children as having no sexual feelings, or having no need of privacy. As he gets better he will want to spend some of his time alone with friends, and this should be respected. Unfortunately, the old friends may not continue to visit, and he will find it hard to meet new friends. Throughout this book we have stressed the importance of professional counselling. This is a time when he needs help. But it is also a time when you as the care-giver could benefit from a sympathetic ear, and benefit from advice about coping with an adult child or friend who is no longer able to manage his own sexual life.

CASE HISTORIES

Michael:

When he no longer spent most of the day asleep, Michael returned to the hospital, where he had been taken immediately after his accident, as an out-patient for the rehabilitation which he needed. Michael spent most time with the speech and language therapist, who worked with him on his reading and writing, as well as giving him exercises to help his poor memory. Michael accepted that he got mixed up with words, and that he forgot things, but he did not enjoy doing activities that in the past would have been simple, but which were now difficult for him. Neither did Michael enjoy discovering that he could not do some of the games and puzzles that the occupational therapist gave him. He made excuses to avoid playing Scrabble, for instance, and sometimes managed to sneak back for some extra work with the physiotherapist rather than do these activities. He was sure that the problems which he had in occupational therapy were because the other patients there were making too much noise, or because the light was wrong, or because the games were not ones that he liked doing anyway.

Michael's mother found things easier with him out of the house for part of the day, but she began to dread his return, because he was so tired that he often was irrational and aggressive. Michael's mother was frightened and worried by these outbursts, but she was reluctant to bother the rehabilitation people with the problem, and she was ashamed to admit to them that her son was so rude to her. Eventually Michael's sister rang their father and insisted that he help.

Michael's father, by now beginning to come to terms with the accident and wanting to make amends for his earlier neglect, arranged for a meeting with the rehabilitation team, so that the family could find out how to cope. It was decided to have Michael stay with his father during the week, so that Michael's mother could have a break. Michael's programme was changed to include more rest periods, so that he did not return home so tired that he could not control his anger. This change also produced an improvement in how he did with his rehabilitation tasks, and he began to appreciate that he did need some help.

Mary:

Six months after the accident Mary still took a long time over everything that she did. Her mother still had her job, and she had worked out a system where Mary's sisters and her father all had their chores to do when they got home, but even so she needed to get up a good two hours earlier than her normal time in the mornings to get things done. Mary's mother was therefore a bit tired and irritable all the time, and she did not cope well when the children squabbled, as they seemed to do often. Mary's sisters resented Mary getting all their mother's attention, and Mary resented not being able to join them in their games and at school. Mary expressed her resentment in physical aggression, and both sisters often sported bite or pinch marks.

Apart from being very slow at doing things, Mary's memory was still not good, and everyone accepted that she was not yet well enough to go back to school. Sometimes her school friends visited her, but these visits became few and far between, because Mary became very excited and giggly when she saw her little friends and they found it hard to know how to act with her.

Arnold:

When it was time for him to return to the hospital for a review, Arnold cancelled the appointment. He told himself that he did not have time to spare sitting around in a waiting room for an hour or so, but the real reason was that he was frightened that he was losing his mind. As time went by, Arnold became more and more aware that something was wrong. He found that he could not cope with problems, and he made some bad decisions, which were expensive and which threatened his reputation as an astute business man. Arnold also found that he had trouble in controlling his emotions, and he was bothered by frequent tears, which to him confirmed the 'nervous breakdown' diagnosis. He had put an end to the relationship with his lady friend, partly because of his wobbly emotions, and partly because he found that he was sexually impotent.

Eventually Arnold realized that he could no longer continue trying to pretend that the accident had not happened, and that he did need to get some professional help. He made and kept an appointment with his general practitioner, an old family friend, and was relieved when his request to be referred to a psychiatrist was met with the explanation that he was not in fact going mad. Although it was difficult, Arnold managed to follow his doctor's advice to stop trying to cope with all his many business affairs and to concentrate on coping with the after-effects of the injury.

6. Some specific consequences

The after-effects of the accident which we talked about in the last chapter can be seen in anyone who has had a closed head injury of the 'acceleration' or 'deceleration' type which we described in Chapter 2, whether this was mild or severe. You will remember that in this sort of injury most parts of the brain are affected by the distortion and twisting which occurs. Penetrating injuries or blood clots, on the other hand, cause a more localized damage, which produces different effects. These are often like the effects of a stroke, as they can cause paralysis of one side of the body, clumsiness and loss of balance, loss of speech, or difficulties in behaviour. Often both sorts of damage are present at the same time and this makes it much more difficult for the victim to overcome the disabilities.

ARMS, LEGS, WALKING, AND BALANCE

All animals, ourselves included, depend on strong, well co-ordinated arms and legs, and a good sense of balance when we are walking or climbing. This is mostly achieved automatically, without thought. Humans have the extra burden of balancing upright, and of controlling skilled movements of the hands and arms. It is no wonder that injury, by accident or disease, has so profound an effect on this complex function.

Weakness

We mentioned in Chapter 2 what is generally known, that damage to one side of the brain commonly results in weakness of the other side of the body, a 'hemiplegia', or 'half-paralysis'. Most people's knowledge of this comes from seeing what happens after a stroke. The hand is usually most affected, and even though other parts recover, the hand will often remain weak and clumsy. Movement at the shoulder and the elbow, and at the hip and thigh, tends to recover more quickly. Although movements may be weak, the muscles themselves are strong, and in many cases are 'spastic', or stiff, so that movement may be automatically resisted. Reflexes may be very active, so that if a muscle is tightened quickly, the calf muscle by putting the foot down on the floor and bending the ankle up, for example, it may contract repeatedly and set up a juddering movement which is called 'clonus'. Over-action of the spastic muscles may pull a joint into an abnormal position where it may stiffen if it is not moved regularly; this is a 'contracture' of the joint. A joint fixed in this position may be a serious handicap to getting function back.

Some head injuries will result in paralysis of this sort, usually those head injuries in which there is a blood clot pressing on one side of the brain and with not much damage elsewhere. In most cases of severe head injury the damage is more widespread, and affects the deeper parts of the brain. This produces a different picture.

In the days immediately after the injury the legs may be stiff and straight, with the toes pointed. The arms will be either straight or sharply bent at the elbow. If the limbs are allowed to stay in this position then stiff contracted joints are common. Later, after some recovery has taken place, one arm and both legs usually remain weak and spastic, the leg on the side of the weak arm being more affected. The other arm can be nearly normal. Many variations may occur in this pattern.

Loss of power in arms and legs

Hemiplegia:
localized damage to one side of the brain
one side of the body affected

Three limbs affected—'triplegia':
widespread damage, including deeper parts of the brain
one arm and both legs affected

Coordination and balance

The ability to co-ordinate arms and legs comes from a different system in the brain. In a stroke, when the damage is confined to one area, very little clumsiness may accompany the weakness. In trauma, which usually produces more widespread damage, co-ordination is likely to be affected along with strength, so that there is both weakness and clumsiness. Occasionally only the co-ordination system is affected, and then there is clumsiness with nearly normal strength.

Balance and a proper posture are other aspects of co-ordination, and are necessary for walking. They depend on several systems in the brain, and each of these may be affected to a different extent. Problems with balance and posture appear in the early stages after a severe injury when the patient first attempts to sit up. Usually his head will fall forward or to the side and his body will slump down. In time muscle tone will improve and he will be able to hold his head up. Then proper tone in the trunk and legs has to be re-learned as he begins to try to stand.

At this stage two other systems come into action. The first makes it possible to recognize what position your body is in and how it relates to the world around. Fit people take this for granted; they know instantly which way is up and with a glance they know what is around them, what they can lean on, what is holding them up, and what they could reach out and touch for support. In many cases this ability is lost after brain injury. Fit people find it difficult to appreciate how frightening this can be; the nearest comparison is living one's life on a roller coaster. The head injury victim needs to re-learn these important skills so that each day his body can get a little more upright and his senses can learn to estimate what is around him.

The other important system is inner ear balance, the 'vestibular system'. The balance organs are enclosed in dense bone at the base of the skull, along with the organs of hearing. They are very small and delicate, and easily upset. Even after mild head injuries there are often balance problems, which show up as a feeling of dizziness and spinning, most often when the head is moved suddenly. Severe injuries are likely to put them out of action altogether, and the lack of information about balance may make it very difficult to sit securely and to make the first moves towards walking.

Co-ordination
Needs strength, but control as well

Balance
Needs co-ordination
Needs information from: balance organs in ears
                       vision
                       experience and thinking

Posture
Needs strength, control, balance, and sustained effort
Necessary in order to begin walking

Much of the early rehabilitation will be taken up with these problems. In the stage of coma the physiotherapists will make sure that joints are kept moving, and at the same time protected from the strains that the abnormal postures of an unconscious person can cause. As consciousness returns, the physiotherapists will start to get the patient sitting up in a chair, at first helping him to hold his head up, then onto a tilting bed to accustom the patient to being upright, and at length standing. In this way he will re-develop the skills of knowing where he is in space and of controlling his posture.

Walking

In getting as far as this, he will have taken a few uncertain steps from bed to chair; now he can start in earnest to re-learn to walk. This is one of the major goals of recovery, a sign of achievement and independence. To begin with support will be needed, from therapists, then from wheeled frames that steady the balance and take some of the weight on the arms, and then from sticks. Splints may be used to strengthen the knee or hold a foot in good position.

How close recovery of walking is to normal will vary, and depends mostly on the severity of the injury. Some will get to walking much as they did before. At the other extreme, they may be able to take only a few steps and prefer to use a wheelchair to get around outside their home. The best measure of success is how good their function is, rather than how close to normal they look. This is an important point because people sometimes become obsessed by the need to walk and reject practical aids to function such as sticks and wheelchairs.

Everyday living skills

At the same time as posture, balance, and mobility are being regained, the occupational therapists will be using these re-learned skills to get the victim back to the business of everyday living. Eating, washing, and all the other simple activities will teach him again to know where he is, what is going on around him, and how he relates to the world. Later, their teaching will extend to improving co-ordination by using manual skills, writing, using a typewriter, and a computer.

Regaining the skills of everyday life
Using re-learned co-ordination and balance to cope with simple
  activities (eating, washing, etc.)
Improving co-ordination and balance by using manual skills

Spontaneous movements

Some people develop troublesome spontaneous movements after a head
injury, which you may hear called 'chorea' or 'ballismus'. Usually just
one arm is affected. Either at rest or in the middle of a movement the arm
will suddenly make a quite inappropriate movement, occasionally quite
violently. The arm usually moves as a whole, but sometimes just the
hand or fingers may be affected. The cause is damage to the deep central
parts of the brain. Medication may help. Sometimes an operation on the
brain, similar to the operation that can be used in Parkinson's disease,
may be advised.

POST-TRAUMATIC EPILEPSY

Diagnosing post-traumatic epilepsy

In Chapter 2 we saw that damage to parts of the brain can result in
scarring which destabilizes the brain and leads to epilepsy. Epilepsy
shows itself by 'fits', or to use the less-distressing term, 'seizures'. There
are several sorts of seizure. Most easily recognized is the major seizure,
in which consciousness is lost and there is to-and-fro shaking of arms and
legs. In other sorts of seizure consciousness may be lost without any
noticeable movements, sometimes for quite a short period and without
much else to see. The victim may fall as the legs give way, or he may
remain standing in the same position. During the seizure or after it is
over he may carry out actions which are quite well organized but inappropriate, such as walking round in a circle, or saying a few words.
He may be confused for a while. Sometimes the seizures may be even less
noticeable, and described as 'just shutting off' for a few moments.

Usually the family will have little doubt that something unusual is
happening, except with the 'shutting off' episodes or the very minor
seizures, and their doctor will be told about it right away. Coming to a
diagnosis about the nature and cause of the seizure will depend very

much on a close description of what happened, and it will be very helpful if family get as detailed a description as they can, preferably writing down what happened.

Usually an electroencephalogram (EEG) is carried out to help to diagnose the cause of the seizure. We mentioned the EEG in Chapter 2; it is a recording of the minute electric currents from the brain, picked up by wires resting on the scalp. It must be emphasized that this technique only helps diagnosis; it is not the last word, and indeed it sometimes may not show any abnormality even though there are definite seizures.

Post-traumatic epilepsy
'Major' seizures with convulsions
'Minor' seizures, 'shutting off'

Diagnosis of seizure
Requires a good description of what happened
EEG recordings, which do not need to be abnormal

Treatment

When a definite diagnosis of post-traumatic epilepsy has been made, 'anticonvulsant' medication will usually be recommended. The medication works by reducing the tendency of the brain to become destabilized by the irritation from the scarring. If it is going to be used at all then it must be taken regularly all the time as a protection, as a sort of insurance policy. There is no point in taking it irregularly, and in fact this may be harmful. If the medication has to be stopped then it must be tailed off gradually over two or three weeks. Stopping it abruptly may set off a seizure.

When the medication is first started it will be necessary to check that the dose is correct. This will be judged by whether it is working, by stopping the seizures, and whether there are any unpleasant side effects. The amount of anticonvulsant in the blood will often be measured as an additional guide. Later, reviews of dosage will be made every six months or so, or if there are more seizures or any side effects.

What is the risk of post-traumatic epilepsy occurring?

The most important factor which determines the chance of contracting post-traumatic epilepsy is what sort of injury there was. In general, injury to the surface of the brain is more important, and so with open wounds involving the brain the risk is high. Bruises of the brain and clots within it are also potent causes. As a very rough guide indeed, a moderately severe open wound involving five or so square centimetres of the surface of the brain will result in a 20 per cent risk of epilepsy. With more details of the damage, the doctor may be able to give a better estimate of the risk.

The seizures can start in the first days or weeks after the accident, or they can appear up to five or more years later. The risk lessens as time passes. After three years it is less than a quarter of the original risk, and after ten years it is probably no greater than the risk in the population as a whole.

Can post-traumatic epilepsy be prevented?

The first measure to prevent epilepsy is to make sure that wounds are treated properly. If the wound is cleaned thoroughly and all damaged tissue removed it will heal smoothly without inflammation and so the risk will be reduced.

The second measure is to give anticonvulsant drugs to try to prevent epilepsy occurring. It is possible that if the drugs are given immediately after the injury then the damaged area never gets a chance to destabilize the brain round it, and that if the drugs are then discontinued after a year or so, the risk is over. It is fair to say that it has not yet been shown whether or not this is the case. However, many doctors think that epilepsy is so disabling that if there is a reasonable chance of reducing the risk then it is worth the inconvenience of taking medication for a year. This is a choice which should be discussed with the patient and family to decide on the merits of each case—how big the risk is and how they feel about taking the precaution.

Treating post-traumatic epilepsy

Medication *should* be started:
when it is certain that seizures are occurring

Medication may be *chosen*:
when the risk of epilepsy is high   (cont.)

Treating post-traumatic epilepsy (cont.)

If medication is being taken:
it must be taken regularly

If medication is stopped for any reason:
it must be tailed off
dosage and levels of drug in the blood must be checked regularly

Stopping anticonvulsant medication

If medication has been given to try to prevent epilepsy, after a year or so the decision will have to be made whether or not to stop it. If seizures have occurred in this period, plainly the medication will have to be kept on.

If there have not been any seizures, the decision may be more difficult. When we discontinue medication we will be waiting to see whether a seizure occurs. For someone who is still in hospital undergoing rehabilitation this is not a great risk. For someone who is out in the community and perhaps driving a car, the decision poses great problems. Should the victim continue to drive, or to go swimming or sailing, accepting the risk that he may have a seizure in a place of danger? Should he avoid doing some activities until he knows if he has epilepsy? If so, how long will he have to wait?

There is no easy answer to our questions. The patient's lifestyle is one of the major factors. How much does he depend on using his car, what is his work, can he come to a reasonable conclusion about this problem, or has his judgement been affected by the accident? The other major factor must be the risk of having a seizure. We can get an estimate of this from the nature of the injury. This estimate can be strengthened by the information from an EEG. Unfortunately if the EEG is normal, it cannot be taken as ruling out epilepsy. If the EEG is definitely abnormal it can be a good reason for continuing with medication, but if there is an objection to this then the alternative is to discontinue it and live a rather restricted life for a year or so to see whether or not a seizure will occur. This is not completely safe, but may be a reasonable thing to do.

When as much of the information as possible has been assembled a final decision must be made by patient and doctor, with the help of the partner or other close relative. If it is decided to discontinue, the drug must be reduced slowly over two or three weeks, and definite safety rules agreed on for the next six months or so, depending on the estimate of risk. If medication is to be continued, another date for review should be set, in perhaps a year.

Stopping medication

Making the decision:

if the victim has never had seizures but has taken medication to prevent them

if the victim has had seizures but with medication has had no more for several years

The decision will depend on:

the risk of more fits: your doctor can give advice about this on the basis of the facts of the injury and on tests such as EEG

how another fit will affect the victim; danger at work, driving and social effects

---

Discontinuing anticonvulsant drugs can also become an issue when they have been started or continued because of seizures and a number of years have passed without any further evidence of epilepsy. There is no doubt that in some people the tendency to seizures does diminish with the years. All the evidence possible of activity of the epilepsy should be gathered, and a decision taken in the light of this and the patient's life-style. Again, there are no easy answers.

LANGUAGE

In most people, the ability to speak is controlled by parts of the left side of the brain. When these parts are damaged speech can be affected in several ways. Other parts of the brain, close to the speaking areas, are needed for us to understand what people are saying to us, and again damage here can affect us in several ways. Further towards the back of the brain, but still in the left half, are the areas that we use when we read, or when we write. The skills of talking, listening, reading, and writing are all different ways of using language. This section looks at what happens when there is damage to these 'language areas'.

Two different names are given to speech problems which result from damage to the special language areas of the brain. These are aphasia (which literally means no speech) and dysphasia (damaged speech).

When the problem is with understanding what has been said, it is called 'receptive aphasia' (if nothing can be understood) or 'receptive dysphasia' if the victims can understand only some of the speech that they hear. The terms 'expressive aphasia' or 'expressive dysphasia' are used to describe problems with producing speech.

Understanding speech

When your friend or relative first wakes up after the head injury he may be confused and muddled, and answers to your questions may not make much sense. This does not necessarily mean that he has damaged the 'listening to speech' areas, however. More probably it is because at this stage he is not properly awake, and he is rather like someone who has over-indulged in alcohol. However, the person with damage to the areas of the brain which are needed for us to understand speech is often as difficult to communicate with as a drunk. Sometimes he is not able to react to any speech at all. More often he will have problems sorting out what different nouns and verbs mean, or he may have difficulty with the small words that link the nouns and verbs together.

You will appreciate that if the victim is to benefit from rehabilitation, he must regain the ability to take in the messages and instructions that he is given. For this reason, intensive work with the speech and language therapist is paramount, and the other members of the rehabilitation team may not be able to start work until the patients have regained some basic communication skills.

Producing speech

There are several different ways that the ability to speak can be disturbed by damage to different parts of the brain. The first is where there is damage to the speech control apparatus, or to the nerves that serve this apparatus. Here the choice of words which are to be said, and the way the words are put together to get the meaning across, are fine. The right words are used, and the words are combined in the right way. The problem is in getting the speech apparatus to produce the sounds. There may be reduced energy, so that only a whisper comes out, or reduced modulation, so that the cadence of the speech is abnormal, or some distortion so that pronunciation of some vowels or consonants is wrong. These problems are usually called dysarthrias and not dysphasias. The problems are the result of disturbance of the production of speech sounds, but these problems do not mean that there has been any disturbance of the ability to understand or use language. For severely disabled anarthric patients, aids such as electronic communicators or word processors may be useful, and may help to give the patients back the ability to get what they want to say across to those around them.

A head-injured victim who has sustained damage to the language production areas is less fortunate. When this damage has occurred, it is usually very obvious. Sometimes he will not be able to say any words at all, although he may be able to make all the isolated speech sounds that are needed. Sometimes he will say a lot of words, but the words will not have any meaning. Sometimes many real words will be used, but the way that they are put together does not always make sense. Sometimes only a few words will be used ('yes' and 'no' are often the only recognizable 'speech words') but they may be used inappropriately. Sometimes the grammar and syntax of the person's speech may be appropriate, but the words that are used are nonsense. Sometimes the person will have problems saying the right naming word, but otherwise speech is normal. In all these cases the problem is in the use of language to communicate.

The problems described may be, and often are, accompanied by corresponding problems with written communication. When they are, the victim is not able to make himself understood by using alternatives to speech such as typing or writing words. You will want to follow the advice of the speech and language therapist who is working with your friend or relative. The therapist will be able to tell you how to help him make himself understood, and how to make it easier for him to understand what you are saying to him.

There are, however, two important points to remember if head-injured people do have language problems. The first is that just because he is not able to express himself, to say any words, does not mean that he is not able to understand what is said to him. Always act as if he understands. If you do this, it will prevent hurtful situations arising where thoughtless visitors make comments in his presence which bother him but which he cannot discuss and about which he cannot make his concern known.

The second point to remember is that emotional language seems to be handled by other parts of the brain than are used for understanding or expressing speech. Emotional language means language such as wearing, which is used mainly to communicate how we feel about something. Because it does depend on different parts of the brain, it can often be used even when the ability to use speech to communicate information is severely affected. Family and friends are often unnecessarily disturbed to hear the victim saying nothing but swear words. Remember that not being able to express himself is even more disturbing to him than it is to you, and that it is his high level of frustration which is evoking the words.

If communication is a problem

Speak slowly and clearly
Use questions that only need yes or no to answer
Keep sentences simple
Always act as if the victim understands what you say

COPING WITH THE WORLD AROUND US

Just as damage to the parts of the brain that are needed for us to use language can affect both understanding of what we hear and also our ability to use speech, so does damage to some parts in the other half of the brain affect both how well we are able to understand what we see, and to interact with the world around us.

Understanding what we see

By the time we have passed childhood we have established many 'seeing' skills which we no longer have to think about. We are able to tell that a square table is square, for example, even when we look at it from an angle so that the eye sees it as a squashed rectangle. We can also make very complicated calculations almost instantly, and without thinking, when we decide how far away something is. We not only use this skill whenever we cope with road traffic, either as driver or pedestrian, but also whenever we reach out to touch something or negotiate our way round obstacles.

Damage, especially to parts towards the back of the brain in the half opposite to that which is used to cope with language, can make it very difficult to use these 'automatic' skills. The victim is usually affected in one of two ways. He may make mistakes in understanding what he sees around him, or he may neglect things which he ought to have seen.

Making mistakes in what the victim sees shows in not being able to tell how far or near things are around him. This obviously makes it unsafe for him to engage in some activities (driving a motor vehicle, for example). It may be difficult for him to re-train the brain to get the right answers. By the time we reach adulthood making judgements about distance has become so automatic that we no longer know how we do it! For the same reason, it is very hard for him to re-learn to interpret or to identify things that he sees.

It is often very difficult for family and friends to understand why the victims do what they do. It is so immediately obvious to the uninjured person that the table is where it is that they cannot understand why a head-injured person is unable to avoid it when he walks, or why in trying to place a cup on the table it falls to the floor. It is even more difficult for them to understand how someone can miss seeing something that is so obviously there to them. Usually people who have had this sort of brain damage will miss seeing things on just one side of them. It is typically the left side which is missed or 'neglected' to use one of the technical terms for this problem. The other term is 'inattention'. Regardless of what words are used to describe the problem it happens not because something is wrong with the victim's eyes, but because something is wrong with the part of the brain that makes sense of what is in the field of vision. We know this because when we draw attention to an object that someone has missed, he will then be able to see it.

If your friend or family member has this problem it will help for you to always place yourself on the good side, away from the side of the body where he is likely to miss things. By doing this you are making it much more comfortable for him to concentrate on you and what you are saying. You should also place things that you want him to have or to handle on this good side.

Do not stand or speak on the side that is neglected

Interacting with things around us

In the last section we explained how some types of damage to the brain make it hard for the victim to understand or to interpret what is seen. Obviously if he has these problems, he will also have difficulty in handling the things that he sees wrongly or misses seeing at all. There can also be difficulties when he has a related problem in using his hands appropriately. In the extreme case, he may not use the affected hand and arm at all. This complete neglect of one arm is not because it is paralysed and cannot move, but it is rather similar to the neglect of things that they 'see' but do not react to. It can be distressing to family and friends because, unless reminded, the victim may not dress the affected side of the body, and appear with only one leg in his pyjama pants or only one arm in a sweater. Fortunately this kind of problem usually only lasts for a short time after the injury.

Problems in getting the arm to move appropriately may last longer. There may be difficulties in using things like scissors, which need co-ordinated movements, or in doing things like eating with a knife and fork, which depend on both hands working together. Allow your relative or friend extra time to carry out these tasks if they are difficult for him. Never take over and do them yourself. He will feel bad enough about not being able to use the arm very well without this extra blow to his self respect! It may help you to feel better about sitting back and not doing things for the victim if you remember that the only way he is going to improve is if he is allowed to keep trying things himself.

OTHER SENSES: TASTE, SMELL, TOUCH, AND TEMPERATURE

Taste and smell

We will talk about taste and smell together because they are closely related, they are damaged together, and they recover together. A large part of our enjoyment of food is in the aroma which comes from the kitchen during its preparation, and a large part of the satisfaction that we get from a meal comes from the taste of the food that we have eaten, so being unable to smell or taste is a significant handicap. The nerves that serve the taste buds on the tongue, and the cells in the nose which carry the sensations of smell, are often put out of action for a while after a head injury. If this is because they have been bruised or squashed then the ability to taste and smell things will come back once they have recovered, although this may take many weeks or months.

No recovery can be expected if the nerves have been torn, and the victim will need to adjust his environment to make this safe for him. His doctor will warn him about things to avoid (using acrylic paints in a confined space, for example) and the occupational therapist will help him to work out ways of doing everyday things safely (using timers when he is cooking to warn him when the food is ready, for example).

Often after a head injury food tastes may change, even though the victim has not lost the ability to taste and smell things. He may, for instance, no longer like coffee, or he may develop an appetite for sweet things, or a particular type of food. This might be because of some change in the way that the nerves for taste and smell now function, although it is more likely that it represents changes in the control areas in the brain.

Temperature

In Chapter 2 we explained how the brain stem is the part of the brain that is responsible for body functions which we do not control consciously. Body temperature is one of those functions. When the brain stem is damaged, temperature control can be less efficient. Sometimes people feel abnormally cold, even in the middle of summer. They may need to use electric blankets or heaters when everyone round them is complaining of the heat, and pile on extra clothes when people around them are down to the minimum. In most cases this sensation of excessive cold is part of the way that the body signals that it is tired. Normal temperature control often returns once the person is no longer fatigued.

Altered temperature control can also be shown in feelings of excessive heat, with exactly the opposite problems to those noted in the last paragraph. Again, it seems to be linked to fatigue, and the extent of the problem varies with the degree of tiredness. Apart from the fact that your friend or relative may attract some odd looks because his clothing is not normal for the season, this problem with temperature control is not life threatening, or something that you need to worry about. Allow the victim to determine the clothing and environment that he needs to be comfortable.

CASE HISTORIES

Michael:

Although the blood clot that Michael had did some damage to the part of his brain which is important in the use of language, most of the time he managed to speak quite easily, and to understand what was said to him. However, it was very obvious when Michael was tired which part of the brain had been hurt because he then got his words mixed up, and sometimes what he wanted to say did not come out the way that he had meant it. The rehabilitation team had warned his parents about this.

The rehabilitation team had also warned Michael's parents that even a small amount of alcohol would affect his speech, and that he should not drink at all. Michael's father made sure that he did not drink in front of him, and was consistent in reminding him of this advice. However, on his girl friend's birthday a group of his university friends took Michael and his girl friend to a cabaret to celebrate. As the celebration progressed, Michael's friends forgot the promise they had made to Michael's father that they would not give him any alcohol, and Michael had a glass or two of beer. The evening came to an untimely end when Michael appeared to be grossly intoxicated, and the management asked that he be taken home.

Michael's friends sobered quickly at this, and realized that they could not take Michael back to his father in that state, so they put him to bed on the couch in one of the student flats to 'sleep it off'. To their horror, while they were continuing with the party he started to twitch and jerk, and lost control of his bladder. As can happen, the alcohol had triggered a seizure. It was a birthday which his girl friend never forgot.

Mary:

Mary continued to avoid jigsaw puzzles and colouring books, but it was not until Mary's mother took her into town for the first time that she realized that this was because she was not able to understand what she saw in the same way as before the accident. The realization came as they waited to cross a busy street. Mary became upset and agitated, and refused to cross if there was a car anywhere in sight. She insisted that the car was too close, even though it was obvious to Mary's mother that there was plenty of time, and that the car was a long way off in the distance. Eventually the only way they were able to get across the road was to make a detour to a light-controlled intersection, where Mary could see the signal to pedestrians to walk.

It was after this experience that Mary's mother began to carry out the rehabilitation therapists' advice to spend time with Mary doing the puzzles and games which she had found difficult. The main reason that she had not followed this advice was not that she did not have much spare time, although this was of course true, but that Mary became upset and threw a tantrum whenever she tried to get her to do these activities. Mary's mother had a meeting with the therapists and explained the difficulty. A retired school-teacher friend willingly accepted the suggestion that she take on the task of playing the games. Mary soon found that her protestations were ignored, and as time went on that she was indeed getting better at the puzzles.

Arnold:

Although Arnold had not had a very severe head injury, he had been hurt badly enough to affect his temperature control. One of the changes which he thought was a sign of mental breakdown was that how hot or cold he felt did not depend so much on the environment that he was in as on how tired he was. On a hot, bright, sunny day he could feel as cold as if it were the middle of winter, for example, if he was tired. Indeed he could sometimes only cope by going off to bed with the electric blanket switched on to high. When he woke he would feel uncomfortably hot, and so on until he tired again.

Once his doctor had explained to him that temperature regulation was a problem which some people can have after a head injury, he did not worry too much about it. However, his daughter was sure that he must be sickening for something when she came to visit him one summer evening and found him wrapped up in his winter woollies. It needed a call from the doctor to convince her that she did not need to worry!

7. Needs of particular groups

Statistics show us that more than 50 per cent of all head-injury cases are young men aged between 17 and 25 years and that the injuries happen in road traffic accidents. The two next largest groups are pre-school children who fall from windows, down stairs, or from playground equipment, and old people who are mostly injured in falls at home. People in these and other special groups can all have the same sorts of problems that were discussed in Chapter 5, but often with important individual variations. This chapter discusses the particular problems that head injury raises for some special categories of people and what can be done to help them. However, remember when you are reading this section that all cases are different. Not all small children will have the problems that we talk about and not all older people will find head injury so difficult to overcome.

THE HEAD-INJURED SMALL CHILD

Small children have special problems after head injury for several reasons. The first is the difficulty which they have in understanding what has happened to them, and in passing on how they feel to their parents. It is unlikely, for example, that their vocabulary will include the words 'headache' or 'dizzy'.

Adults who have had a head injury often have difficulty with self-control, and they may express this with physical aggression. A child is only just beginning to learn self-control, so it is not surprising that tantrums are common after the accident, and that injury to itself and to others can occur. Parents will notice that the child's behaviour is worse when he is tired, and they need to make sure that he has plenty of rest. They should watch the child carefully, and as soon as he shows signs of irritability he should be put to bed for an extra sleep. Other strategies which can help are to make sure that there are plenty of different activities available to keep the child's interest, and to give him a chance to work off his irritability with physical exertion, such as bouncing on a trampoline.

Parents will find that caring for a head-injured small child involves almost 24-hour supervision, and this is too much to expect from any person. If the problem lasts for any length of time then the parents need to make sure that there are relatives or friends who can help, to give them some time for themselves and for the other children.

The next reason why head injury at this age is a special problem is that the pre-school years are the time when a tremendous amount of learning takes place. By the time children are three or four they have not only acquired the basic skills of walking and manipulating with their hands, but they can express simple concepts in speech, recognize what they see, and make simple comparisons. All of this depends on an effective memory but, as we have seen, this ability is very likely to be damaged in a head injury.

What does this mean for the child? Fortunately, the skills that he has already mastered are likely to be retained, although he may have some difficulty in using them because of other factors such as fatigue and irritability. From the time of the accident, however, the child may have greater difficulty in building on those skills, and he may progress more slowly than his peers. This is a cumulative process. If the accident occurred at a time when the child would normally be acquiring the ability to tell the difference between various shapes and angles, he will then find it difficult to tell the difference between letters making up a word. If the child then has difficulty in learning to read, he will fail in the next step of education, and so on.

Small children

May not be able to explain how they feel

May not be able to control irritability

May be restless and aggressive

May not learn well

May fall behind their peers

What can you do to help? A clue comes from what happens when head injury or some other condition damages the part of the brain that controls talking and language. Although to begin with speech may be lost completely, most children manage to understand speech and talk again quite quickly. Partly this is because the brain of the small child is not as 'specialized' as that of an adult, and it seems to be easier for other areas of the brain to take over the control of speech. Another reason why speech is regained may be that the child gets plenty of practice listening to words after he has had an accident. Parents and friends amuse the child with stories, as special treats because he has just come home from hospital, and he continually hears family members talking between themselves. We have seen that constant repetition is the basis of rehabilitation techniques, and it may be that the constant exposure to speech which a child who has been in hospital is subjected to is a kind of informal rehabilitation procedure.

It is possible that children may be taught in the same way, by constant repetition, to regain other skills which they have lost. Many children's games and activities are good practice for visual and perceptual abilities. Ask your child's pre-school teacher or occupational therapist to suggest puzzles which may help.

THE HEAD-INJURED SCHOOLCHILD

Although the older child will already have established the language and visual skills needed to read and write, impaired memory will still be a handicap because the school years are obviously a period when the ability to learn is important. We know that the child might have problems with new subjects, such as learning a second language, and it is sensible to delay French lessons, for example, until memory is a little better. We also know that often a child who has had a severe head injury cannot remember some of the schooling that he has already done (this is because of the 'retrograde amnesia' described in Chapter 5). It is unfair to expect children to learn a particular level of mathematics if they have no memory for the previous time at school when the basics which are needed to cope with that level were covered. In this case it is sensible to put off the higher maths lessons, and to go over the learning that has been 'lost'.

It is not just the learning difficulty that a child may have after head injury which is a problem for them. The typical classroom with one teacher to up to thirty or so children is not an easy environment for any child to cope with after a head injury. A head-injured child will have concentration problems, so he will find it hard to keep his attention on the lesson and to ignore the many distractions in the room. He will probably take longer to do things, so he will not be able to finish his work in the same time as the other children. He will tire more quickly, and as he gets tired his concentration will deteriorate even further, and he is likely to become restless and labelled as having 'behaviour problems'.

It is easy to see how the child can be seen by his classmates and his teachers as naughty and/or stupid, even though before his accident his behaviour and achievement level may have been average or better. It is an unfortunate fact that children can be blunt and unkind in their reactions to others who are different in some way, and it often is impossible for the head-injured child to live down the 'dummy' label which was given at this stage. The issue of managing return to school after head injury is covered more fully in Chapter 9. Here it is important to remember that the need for the child to have contact with his peers has to be balanced against the importance of making sure that he has recovered sufficiently to cope with this contact without destroying his self-confidence.

Parents and care-givers are sometimes better able to estimate the staying power of their child and how much should be expected of him than are the rehabilitation staff, who may only work with the child for a few hours each week. However, as well as this information about how much the child can do before he tires, we also need to know how good his memory is, how fast his reaction times are, and how well he can concentrate, before we can reach a sensible decision about starting back at school. This is the sort of information that we can get from a good objective assessment carried out by an experienced rehabilitation specialist. This information will be used in guiding the return to school, and it is important to stress that this will not be started before the child is ready, neither will it be delayed after he has regained sufficient ability to cope.

What about the child who was already having problems at school before the accident? Well, we can be very sure that the head injury is not going to cure these problems. It is less easy to decide whether or not school is going to be even harder for the child. If the head injury was very severe, your doctor will be more definite about the need to expect problems than if it was relatively minor. But in either case do make sure that you get advice about the process of returning to school. It also helps if the child can return to a school that is familiar to him, and to teachers who have taught him before.

We have talked mainly about the problems the older schoolchild has with learning, and with getting back into the school system. There are other problems. Time does not stand still, and as the months and then years since the accident slip past, younger brothers and sisters continue to grow and develop, and often to overtake the head-injured child in social skills as well as in education. However secure and well-adjusted he may seem to be, the teen-age victim of a head injury will find it hard to be happy about a younger sibling starting to date before him, or succeeding on the sports field where he never could. Counselling, to help your child come to grips with the effects of the accident, may have been offered earlier on. Sometimes it is important to have counselling at a later stage also, and the child often is more receptive when events, such as seeing a younger brother do the things that they cannot do, bring home the reality of the accident to them.

There is indeed a good case to be made for counselling, or at least advice, to be given every six months or so to family, to friends, and to teachers. In the early stages after the injury no one needs reminding about the accident or the way it has affected the patient. As time goes by it is sometimes less obvious that the child has been injured and that he still has problems. Indeed there may be overt comments like 'But the accident was years ago: he must be recovered by now' when it is suggested that the victim still cannot cope with a normal daily programme. As we point out in the next chapter, families often expect recovery to follow the same sort of pattern in everyone, and find it difficult to cope with the concept that the degree of recovery and the time it takes is uncertain. Regular counselling would also help parents to cope with the problems which may develop as their child grows into adolescence with a disability.

THE HEAD-INJURED ELDERLY PERSON

By the time people reach their sixth or seventh decade they will probably have found that they are more forgetful, a bit slower, and perhaps not quite as efficient as when they were younger. Certainly they will know that in matters of judgement and 'wisdom' they are in their prime, but they would probably hesitate to challenge a younger person to a competition which required making quick decisions. This is an inevitable, and normal, part of ageing. So already, even before the accident, the elderly head-injured victim has probably experienced some of the after-effects of a head injury to some degree. Thus it is not surprising that an older person usually is more incapacitated, and does not recover as quickly, or as completely, as someone in their teens or twenties. Yet the victim is at an age when his years of experience often mean that he is at the peak of his career.

There are advantages and disadvantages to having an important position at work. The victim may insist that he cannot take time off work because he is needed to run the ship, as it were. Or he may worry that he will lose his position of authority to his juniors if he is away too long. So he runs a real risk of returning to work before he has recovered well enough to cope with the work, and of failing. This puts a tremendous strain on the family, who find themselves in the position of having to tell father or mother that he or she is not good enough any more to handle the jobs which he or she have maybe done for a quarter of a century. And if, as so often happens, the elderly person does not have much insight into the head-injury problems, the family also have the task of correcting errors and picking up the pieces.

If your head-injured relative or friend falls into this age-group, you will know by now that you can need as much help and support as he does. Pride may make it hard for you to let friends, or even other family members, realize how much he has changed. Pride may also make it hard for you to ask for help. If professional counselling is available then take advantage of it. In these cases it is usually easier to unburden your fears to an outsider.

We said that the fact that the elderly person has reached the peak of his career also has its advantages. One advantage is that he has no doubt learned some ways of compensating for the decline in memory that has crept up over the years. He has already learnt that he has to use the diary, the calendar, and the other memory aids which we talked about in Chapter 5. The other advantage is that often he is in a position to re-organize his role to that of advisor or mentor, and often can restrict the hours of work to those he can manage. Provided he is aware of the limitations that he has, he can modify his lifestyle so that the demands he makes of himself fall within his capacity at that stage.

It may be, however, that the best option is to take early retirement, and to use these extra years to develop a hobby or activity that there was never enough time for up until now. It is often more realistic to accept that the years of paid employment are over than to struggle to achieve the goal of 'return to work' when this is simply going to lead to frustration and disappointment. Your support as the carer will be very important at this stage, and you also will need to accept that this is a positive step which will make your own life, and that of the head-injured victim, much less difficult.

> After head injury an elderly person is unlikely to recover as quickly or as completely as a younger person

So far we have concentrated on the elderly person who was still in the work force at the time of injury. People who have already retired may also have to make changes to their lifestyle, and these will often affect their independence. If your relative or friend lives alone and if memory and concentration problems put him at risk, for instance of burning his house down, it will be necessary to make arrangements for his safety. Your circumstances may be such that you can have your relative or friend to live with you, but you should remember that older people do not recover either as quickly or as completely as the young, and that the arrangement may turn out to be a permanent one.

THE HEAD-INJURED PSYCHIATRIC PATIENT

People with a history of psychiatric disorder can, like anyone else, suffer a head injury. If the person you are caring for comes into this category, it may be harder for him to deal with the head injury.

The general effects of the head injury may be very similar to those of his illness, such as tiredness, poor concentration, aggression, and mood changes. Because of his illness he may have less ability to deal with the more specific head-injury problems such as headache and dizziness or disabilities of movement, speech, and thought. Also, head injury symptoms, such as the sleep disturbance that may occur, can make his psychiatric condition worse. Medication that a psychiatric patient needs may slow down his reaction times and affect his ability to concentrate, and the tests used to assess mental function after head injury may become misleading. It may therefore become very difficult to decide which condition is responsible for the symptoms he shows. Because you know him well, you may be able to do this better than the rehabilitation team, and thus be a great help to them. You can let them know the ways in which he has changed, and the things that were a problem to him even before the accident. You will also know the sorts of things that he responds to, and how *not* to treat him.

We have stressed the importance of support and counselling for carers and family members. You need to have the chance to talk with other people who have had relatives with similar problems. Sometimes this can be arranged through your local head-injury organization, and sometimes there will be someone in a psychiatric support group who can give you this help. In either case, while you have the task of caring for someone with both a disorder and an injury, you do need to use any agency that is available to provide a 'minder' for the victim, so that you can have some time to yourself and to spend with the other members of the family.

THE HEAD-INJURED SUBSTANCE ABUSER

A substance abuser has similar difficulties to the patient who has a history of psychiatric illness in that he has problems which existed before the head injury which often make it hard for the rehabilitation team to decide what effect the accident has had. In addition, if the victim has been taking drugs or alcohol for some time, he is likely to have had a damaged brain even before the injury, and as with the elderly patient, he is not likely to recover as quickly or as fully as someone who did not have this history.

A substance abuser is likely to have broken away from the family before the injury. In many cases, however, parents or spouses will still feel that they have a responsibility to be the care-giver, and will sometimes see the accident as a time to make a fresh start. Unfortunately this is usually doomed to disappointment.

While the victim is still recovering from a head injury, he will not be able to cope with the demands of a substance abuse programme. You will recall from Chapter 5 that at this stage concentration will probably be poor, the victim is likely to be irritable, restless, aggressive, and he will have difficulty coping with more than one person at a time, and so on. Equally importantly, he will probably have a poor memory and so will not remember what has happened from one session to the next. He may have poor self-control also, so that he cannot be expected to be responsible for his own behaviour. It is unrealistic to expect to get him off the habit now that you have him back. It is also unrealistic to expect that recovery will follow the typical pattern of other head-injured people. There are likely to be withdrawal symptoms and other unpleasant effects, and it is important that he has professional care during this stage.

Unfortunately, because of his lifestyle and the effects which his activities have on his ability, substance abusers are very likely to have falls, fights, and traffic accidents. It is equally unfortunate that, because of the special problems which the substance abuser has, he does not usually do well in rehabilitation. Again this is an area where you may need some professional counselling so that you come to terms with the fact that your help may not be enough to change him.

In terms of the number of people who have a head injury, the sub-groups of children, the aged, the psychiatric or the substance-abuse patients, make up only about half of all cases. Most head-injury patients are young adult males. But again, although the head injury has the potential to damage the same basic physical or cognitive functions in each case, the way these affect the person can be different depending on his role.

THE HEAD-INJURED WOMAN

Even in this last quarter of the twentieth century, in spite of feminism and equal opportunities, expectations of the sexes can be rather different. The 'Big boys don't cry, only girls cry' edict is by no means dead. If your head-injured friend or relative is a woman she is at risk of having genuine complaints of headache and fatigue treated more lightly than if she were a man. She may also find that emotional changes, and weeping frequently, can be ascribed to her sex rather than to the accident. Worse still, she may believe this herself, and think that she is going through a nervous breakdown. You can reassure her. Men and women are different, but the effects of a head injury are present regardless of sex.

Many women also fill the traditional role of home-makers. Few societies recognize this as an occupation in the sense that paid employment is an occupation. Yet the job is probably more demanding and with worse working conditions than any other. What union would allow its members to work, or be on call, for 24 hours a day seven days a week? What union would allow its members to carry out any number of un-specified tasks on demand; tasks as diverse as nursemaid, cook, gardener, and handyman. Home-makers accept this as part and parcel of bringing up a family, and families expect that the home-maker will be on call to do anything for them at practically any time.

What happens when the home-maker has had a head injury? You will have brought her home from hospital probably earlier than would have been the case if she had a 'proper' job waiting for her. She will find it difficult to accept that her role is now to be the cared-for rather than the care-giver. She may see the family doing her job rather incompetently, or at least in a different way from her own. She will also see that her children are not only sad and upset at her accident, but that they often have had to interrupt their schooling or careers to look after her. It is a complete role reversal for the family. Offspring have to comfort and guide the parent and partners have to assume the home-maker as well as the bread-winner role.

It is not surprising that the victim will resist attempts to get her to rest, and she will try to pick up the threads of her normal life again. In the early weeks after she comes home, while the accident is still fresh in your mind, you will find it easy to remember that she needs help. But as time goes by, especially if she looks as well as she did before the accident, it will be easy to slip into the expectation that she also will be able to cope as well as she did then.

THE HEAD-INJURED PARENT

We have talked about some ways in which a head injury affects the female patient. Obviously there are also role changes for any parent who has had a head injury. It is difficult for adult offspring to adapt to the change in role that this brings about. It is even more difficult if the offspring are still young.

Parents usually guide, criticize, and attempt to regulate the behaviour of their children. After a head injury, when their own behaviour may be socially inappropriate (for example, when they may laugh at the wrong time, or say what they think without worrying about the consequences), it is the children who have to do the monitoring. Younger children may be too embarrassed to bring their friends home after school, or fall into the habit of avoiding the head-injured parent because they do not know how to deal with the aggressive or irritating behaviour. Older children may also avoid coming home, or they may make the situation worse by over-reacting to what is seen as unwarranted attacks by the head-injured parent.

The uninjured parent is in the unenviable situation of attempting to act as referee, to hold the family together. However this parent reacts, either the children or the partner may feel that sides are being taken. It is very important not to let this type of adversarial situation develop. If it is your father who has a head injury, remember that he still sees his role as being a parent. You do not stop being his child just because of the accident. What you and your uninjured parent need to do is to build up a system where you can protect him from making costly or dangerous mistakes, but which allow him to maintain his dignity as an adult. He is not a child, so do not treat him as one.

It is tempting to think that family counselling will make things right. Family counselling should help you and the other parent cope with the situation, but it is unlikely to change the head-injured parent. He does not need to be counselled about his role as a parent. The problem is that he knows his role, but cannot, because of the accident, carry out the functions of a parent at this stage.

THE HEAD-INJURED PARTNER

In a relationship where one partner has a head injury, it is the uninjured partner who carries most of the burden for keeping that relationship together. We have talked about role changes in this chapter. This is inevitable, because the effects of head injury prevent the victim from functioning in the way he did before the accident. Probably the most dramatic role change occurs where one member of a partnership has had a severe head injury.

Where the fit partner assumes the role of care-giver, the relationship becomes more akin to that of a parent and a child. The carer may still love the head-injured partner dearly, but as time goes by the responsibility for the care of the head-injured person can change this to a love which is more like that of a parent than a partner. This change will be fuelled by the inability of the victim to react in the same way as before the accident. Each time the victim is irritable, aggressive, or acts in an unreasonable way, their partner becomes more deeply entrenched in the role of a parent with the responsibility for correcting this behaviour.

Another barrier to the resumption of the old relationship is that sexual function is often disturbed after a head injury. In the early stages after discharge from hospital the head-injured person may tire too quickly to do anything but sleep when he gets to bed. There may also be physiological or hormonal changes which interfere with sexual activity. Even where the partnership was very sound, inability to have sexual relations puts a strain on both partners. The less robust partnership may well founder.

THE PERSON WITH A MILD HEAD INJURY

Paradoxical as it may seem, the person who has been unconscious for only a few minutes, and who was not badly injured enough to need to be admitted to hospital, may have as many problems as the severely injured victim who did not regain consciousness for many weeks. This is because it is usually very obvious to those around him that the latter has been badly injured, and he is not expected to be able to do everything which he did before the accident as well as he did it then. A mildly-injured person, however, probably has nothing to show that he has been injured, and so there is unlikely to be visible evidence that he has not recovered from this injury.

For the majority of these cases, this is only a temporary problem, and the victim will get back his ability to concentrate, to remember, and to think quickly in just a few weeks. However, we know that 5-10 per cent will take much longer than that to recover, and that they can be disabled for many months. This slower than normal recovery is a special problem because people in this group have not usually spent more than a few hours in hospital and so they do not have access to rehabilitation programmes, even where these exist. In Chapter 4 we described how a follow-up appointment is usually given to a victim who has spent some time in hospital after a head injury, to check his progress, and we pointed out that this sort of system would be impractical for less severe injuries because of the sheer numbers involved.

There should be a system, however, where people who are likely to be at special risk after a mild head injury can be screened, and which can provide facilities for checking people who continue to have problems. For example, Accident Department personnel need to know that older people, as well as students and those who are in demanding jobs, should be referred for assessment of memory, concentration, and other problems that can follow closed head injury (see Chapter 5) before they get back to work or school. This assessment should be carried out a week or ten days after the accident, by which time the early unpleasant effects, such as nausea and sleeping all the time, should have passed.

Often, understanding the reason for the problems which he has, and a bit of advice about how to cope with them, is enough to carry the mildly-injured person through this stage. Some find that the opportunity to interact with other people who have the same problems is also useful. If your relative or friend is one of the number of people who is taking a while to recover after a minor head-injury then talk with your family doctor about referring them for this help.

CASE HISTORIES

Michael:

In spite of the set-back when he had the seizure, Michael continued to improve. He was well aware that if he was to return to university he would need to be able to study and to remember what he had read, and he was bothered that he still had so much trouble with his memory.

Michael's parents were also concerned that in spite of his concentration being so much better, and his moods less of a problem, he continued to forget what he had heard or read as soon as he moved on to something else. One day while Michael's mother was leafing through a magazine an advertisement caught her eye. The article was headed 'Students, are you bothered by your memory?' and continued with the claim that Dr X's system guaranteed to train anyone to remember everything that they wanted to. It was rather expensive, but Michael's mother felt that this was the answer to her prayers for Michael, and so she posted off the mail order coupon. The memory system turned out to be a set of exercises similar to those Michael was already doing in therapy, and a selection of mnemonic tricks, some of which were well beyond Michael's memory capacity. One needed to have a normal memory in order to learn the tricks designed to make one's memory work better. Because Michael's memory was not normal, the system was a disappointing and expensive failure.

Mary:

Mary had become more and more persistent in her demands to go back to school. Mary enjoyed the sessions with the old school teacher, but missed her friends once their visits had tailed off. She also became more difficult at home, and her sisters had taken to spending time after school with their own friends, and put off returning home as long as they could. Mary's mother was sad for Mary, but Mary's mother was also worried because she had been warned that she would lose her job if she did not manage to be more punctual, and more consistent in her attendance. The rehabilitation team were aware of the problems, and the social worker managed to find a voluntary helper to get Mary ready in the mornings, and to be on hand to look after her when she had had a bad day and was unable to go to the hospital.

The team arranged for Mary to spend some time at a special school for learning-disabled and physically-handicapped children. This turned out to be an unwise decision as Mary was hurt and depressed at being classed, as she saw it, as 'mentally handicapped'. Getting Mary to go there each morning became more of a problem, until reluctantly the special school idea was dropped. At once Mary became much more co-operative; it was as if she was determined not to behave in any way that might imply she needed the special school.

Arnold:

Six months after his accident Arnold was still bothered by many of the after-effects of head injury. He still tired very quickly, and he got flustered if he had to do anything complicated, or finish something within a time limit. By this time Arnold had returned to the hospital for out-patient rehabilitation, and he appreciated the regular contact and reassurance which he got. He had accepted that it would take him longer to recover than if he had been in his teens or twenties. What he found hard to accept was that he could not make plans for his business affairs because he did not know when he would be fit enough to take the reins again.

Eventually, on the advice of his solicitor and accountant, Arnold made the most sensible decision that he had made since his accident. He sold his property company and his restaurant while they still had some market value. Arnold spent an exhausting month with the parts of the negotiations where he had to be present, and left the rest to his advisers. He was pleasantly surprised at the relief he felt when the sales were concluded and the responsibility was taken off his shoulders.

Arnold decided to spend part of the sale proceeds on a holiday, and he persuaded his former lady friend to accompany him to a tropical resort, where they lazed in the sun for a month and re-established their relationship.

8. How long will it take for the patient to recover?

If you break an arm or a leg in an accident your doctor can usually tell you, to within a few days, how long you will need to be in hospital, for how long you will need to wear a plaster cast, and often how long it will be before you will be able to go back to work. If you also received a head injury in that accident most of these predictions become invalid.

Perhaps the most common complaint that families of a head-injured person make about hospitals and hospital staff is that no one can give them a definite answer to questions such as 'Will the patient live or die?' or 'When will the patient get better?' We have already explained in Chapter 3 that this is because the real answer to these questions is often 'We do not know yet. We will have to wait and see'. Although there are sophisticated machines and procedures to monitor brain function, these are never able to give a definite answer about how well someone will recover from a severe head injury. Many of you will have been warned that there is a possibility that your relative or family member might die, or at least become a 'vegetable'. It should be a matter of delight when neither of these events occurs. Instead, a more favourable outcome is often taken as evidence that 'they do not really know anything about head injury'. The fact is that 'they' do, and all the information which was available at that stage showed that there was a possibility of a poor, or no, recovery.

Given that in the early stages after injury it is not always possible to be definite about whether a patient is going to live or die, it is not surprising that many other questions about recovery are also difficult to answer. This chapter looks at some of the most common 'when' and 'how' questions.

WHEN WILL THE PATIENT WAKE UP?

Two different ways are used to describe the stage where a patient is 'asleep' after a head injury. These are that they are 'in a coma' or that they are 'unconscious'. Both mean the same thing although the coma description is the more usual. We have described the ways that your friend or family member is constantly watched while he is in a coma and how there is sometimes regular monitoring of the electrical activity of the brain. As long as there are no changes in these recordings it will usually not be possible for your doctor to tell you how long it will be before the patient will wake up. When there are changes, you may hear the word 'lightening' used. This simply means that the patient is in a less deep coma. In other words, he has already started to react to more things around him. However, it still might take days or weeks for him to move out of the 'coma' stage.

Do not expect a patient to open his eyes, stretch out his arms, and say 'Where am I?', as patients often do in movies or books. People rarely move abruptly from being in a coma to being properly awake. When the patient first starts to take notice of things around him he is likely to be quite confused about where he is and why he is there. He is likely to ask you again and again what happened to him, or why you have not been to see him before, even though you may have spent almost every waking hour at the hospital for many weeks! At this stage he is starting to 'wake up', but he is still not able to remember things that happen to him, probably from one minute to the next. Do not be alarmed, therefore, if the reaction to you is the same again after you have left the room briefly, perhaps to check something with the nurse, or when you return to visit at the start of a new day. Neither should you be alarmed if he appears to have 'lost' several years of life and insists that he is still at school, for example. We described in Chapter 5 how the memory of things that happened both before and after the accident is always disturbed for a while when there is a closed head injury.

Like the stage where the person is unconscious, or in a coma, this stage in which he is confused, repeats himself, and forgets things might last for a short time only, or for days, weeks, or months. It is clear that he is not properly awake, and we compared it to sleep-walking in Chapter 5. So you see that to answer the question of when the patient will wake up, your doctor would need to be able to predict not only how long he will be unconscious, but also how long this confused stage will last. Thus there are two 'when' questions. However, when your relative or friend is past the coma stage, your doctor will have a better idea about how long the next stage will go on for. This is because the confused state usually lasts longer the longer the period of coma has been. This rule of thumb does not allow your doctor to give you the day and date when the patient will 'wake up'. The doctor can tell you things like 'He will probably be like this for a few months yet', or 'He will probably be more aware of things in a few days'; beyond this you simply have to accept the 'wait and see' advice.

These periods of changed consciousness are a time when you, even more than the hospital staff, can help your relative or friend wake up a bit more. You can tell them what music he liked, what his interests were, what he liked to be called. You can bring photos and mementoes in to the hospital ward to remind him of his real life. It is your voice that he will recognize and which is familiar to him, not the voices of the nurses and doctors. Also, you will probably spend more time with the victim each day than any one member of the hospital staff, so you can be an important observer to watch out for changes in the things that he can do.

The hospital staff may suggest to you that you keep a daily journal of this period. Not only will this give you something to do while you are waiting for the patient during the frequent naps that he will take, but also it will be a valuable record for the days and weeks ahead. It is only natural that there will be times when you feel very down and depressed about things, especially when you cannot see much progress from one day to the next. These are the times to get out your diary and remind yourself of how he was only a month or two back, and to realize how much improvement there has been since then. Your relative or friend will also appreciate your work because, as we explained in Chapter 5, he is unlikely to remember anything of the early weeks when he was in hospital. Later on, when he is able to, he will read about what you and he went through.

WHEN WILL THE PATIENT WALK AND/OR TALK?

In Chapter 6 we described how some patients may be paralysed, or have problems with balance and walking for a while after the accident. Others may have trouble making themselves understood when they talk. Because every accident is different, and every person who has an accident is different from every other, it is usually impossible for the doctor or therapist who is looking after your relative or friend to answer these questions. The doctor or therapist will be able to tell you about any progress, and will probably do this without being asked because they are also excited about improvement in the patients they are working with.

The problem for you is that while your relative or friend is in the 'Head-Injury Ward' you will have seen many other patients at different stages of recovery. You will have talked to their family members about their accidents and when they happened, how the victims were affected. They will have told you how long it was before they managed to do different things. Why is this a problem? It can be a problem if this leads you to expect that your relative will recover in the same time. It is tempting to assume that because somebody's son is the same age as yours, and has had the same sort of accident, they will start to walk again after the same number of weeks. There are many things which influence how quickly or how fully your relative will recover, including the way the brain was injured in the accident. Again you just have to wait and see, and take things one day at a time.

This does not mean that you should not talk with other families in the ward. It is very important that you do. Even your closest friends or relatives will not understand what you are going through as well as someone who is in the same situation as you are. Many wards will arrange for you to meet with other people who have had a head injury in the family, and many areas now have voluntary agencies which run support groups for families (Appendix B gives contact addresses for those in the UK, USA, and Australasia). The point we are making here, and it is something that the other people at the support groups will tell you also, is that you cannot use the recovery pattern and recovery times of any other patient to judge how long your own head-injured relative or friend will take to recover the same skills.

WHEN WILL THE PATIENT LEAVE HOSPITAL?

Even though you know that the answer to this question will probably be the same as to the others—that is, we need to wait and see—there are some instances when you need to have a more definite answer. One consequence of an extended period in hospital after a head injury is that the person has been removed from his normal home and family life, without having had any chance to prepare for such a prolonged absence from home and work. Yet, until he recovers full consciousness, he will not be able to cope with the effects of this absence.

Following the accident the family has to make many practical decisions for the head-injured person. Rent and mortgages continue to come due whether the home is occupied or not. Should you sublet the flat, give up the lease, sell the house, or put in tenants? Employers have a right to expect that their employees will arrive for work each day. Should you ask the employer to hold the job, to put in a temporary replacement for him, or to accept his resignation? To make these decisions you need to have some estimate about the length of time the person will be in hospital. Usually these issues arise when there has not been very much progress for some weeks after the accident. When you explain the problems to your doctor, he or she will usually be able to advise you, even if he or she cannot tell you exactly how long your relative will be in hospital.

The next most important staff member for you to talk to is the Social Worker. This person will know who to get in touch with in the community, either to put things on hold, or to help you make financial and other arrangements. If your relative is an adult you will find that most countries have quite stringent rules that must be followed before you can use his bank accounts, alter contracts that he has entered into, or sell his property for him. This legislation was developed to protect people from the unscrupulous, and although you may find it rather offensive that anyone could consider that you would not act in the best interest of the head-injured person, it is important to go through the necessary steps if he is likely to be in hospital for an extended period.

WHEN WILL THE PATIENT BE BETTER?

The more time which has passed since the accident, the more information your doctor will have about the kind of injury which your relative has had, and the more the doctor will be able to tell you about how much better he is likely to get, or in less severe cases, when he is likely to have recovered. We have already seen that once the doctor knows how long the patient has been unconscious, he or she will be able to give you some idea about how long the period of confusion will last.

These two after-effects of the accident, coma and the period of confusion and disturbed memory, are used as one of the ways of describing how serious a head injury has been. Generally, the longer the person has been unconscious, and the deeper the stage of coma when he reaches the hospital after the accident, the more badly he has been hurt. Information about how long the 'sleep-walking' stage lasts also gives a clue to how serious the injury has been. Obviously, the worse the injury the longer the patient is going to take to recover, and the less complete this recovery is likely to be.

These two measures can only give an estimate, an educated guess, about recovery and recovery times in any one patient. It is true, in general, that someone who has been in a deep coma for six months will make a less complete recovery than someone who has been unconscious for an hour. But there are some individual cases who make a better or faster than predicted recovery, and others who do worse than expected.

We have stressed that prediction becomes more accurate the more time which has passed since the accident, and the more information there is about how much the patient can do. By the time the person leaves hospital he will have recovered the ability to breathe for himself, move about more or less on his own, and communicate with other people, even if his talking is a little slurred or hesitant. He will be able to dress and feed himself, and manage his own toilet. He may still be a long way from being completely recovered, however.

How information builds up about the injury

How deep is the coma?
How long does the coma last?
How long does the 'sleepwalking' last?
How many physical problems are there?
How well do attention and memory work?
How quickly are problems improving?

Chapter 5 describes some of the problems which the patient may have at this stage. These problems can give you some clues as to how quickly he will get better. If the ability to concentrate is very poor, for example, this will affect everything he does. He will not remember things very well because his attention wanders, he will not progress as well with outpatient therapy because he cannot keep his attention on what he should be doing, and he does not practise the exercises at home because he forgets about them. In short, if his concentration is still very poor when he leaves hospital then he will take longer to recover than someone whose concentration is only mildly affected.

One of the important things about being able to answer the 'When will the patient be better?' question is to know how many of the after-effects of head injury the patient has, and how severe these effects are. Then, of course, your doctor will need to know how quickly these after-effects are improving. This is why your relative or friend will be tested quite often after he has left hospital. Knowing how quickly he is im-proving will allow your doctor to give you some idea of when your relative will be better, but again it will only be an informed guess.

There are many other things apart from how serious the injury was which influence how quickly the patient will recover. One of the most important is further damage to the brain. This might happen if the patient knocks his head again in another accident, or if he uses alcohol or other drugs which have an effect on the brain. It will obviously take longer to recover from one accident if the brain is continuously being injured.

Another factor which affects how quickly the victim will recover is what he does while he is waiting to 'get better'. We know that people who have had a head injury are often not able to cope with stress very well, and if your relative is anxious or worried about things—his job, money, relationships, or his own health—he will most likely not be able to relax, or to get enough sleep, and sometimes he may appear to be getting worse. It is important that you talk with your doctor about this, because this situation often can be helped with stress management programmes or with mild relaxants.

As you might expect, how quickly a patient will get better also depends on what kind of rehabilitation is available for him. We know that he will get better faster if he can get into a head-injury facility where he can be given a fully-structured programme, alternating activities and rest according to his needs, and which will provide an environment where he is not likely to do further injury to the brain, or to develop stress reactions. We also believe that damaged skills will not recover unless they are practised, and this applies to the skill of remembering something that is said to you as much as it applies to the skill of moving a muscle. So there are suitable conditions where recovery is more likely to take place, and to take place more rapidly.

Recovery depends on

The severity of the injury
Whether there is further brain damage
Minimizing stress
Effective rehabilitation
Management of return to work/school

This section has dealt mainly with people who will make a fairly good recovery eventually. They are the people who can be expected to return to work or to school. How this is managed also affects how well and how quickly they will recover. In the next chapter you will find suggestions to help make the move back into the work-place or school as smooth and trouble-free as possible. Finally, there are some people, such as the elderly, who are less likely to make a speedy recovery. These special groups were discussed in Chapter 7.

We have seen that there are several things, apart from the injury, that determine how quickly your relative will get better. To some extent these factors are also important in answering the next question, which is about those people who are unlikely to ever make a full recovery.

HOW MUCH RECOVERY CAN BE EXPECTED?

Almost without exception you can be sure that your relative or friend will be better, sometime in the future, than he is today. How much better he will be is another matter.

We do not expect people who have lost a limb in an accident to grow another one. We know that the disability is permanent, even though a very good artificial limb might be fitted to help compensate for the missing limb. With this sort of aid, a person is able to do most of the things that he could before the injury. Brains are different. Although we know that a person who has damaged parts of his brain will never regenerate them, we do not have any replacement for these areas. Yet in spite of this, we know that the patient can quite often get to do some of the things that a particular bit of the brain controlled. How can this happen?

Sometimes it is because the bit of the brain which is needed to allow the patient to do the activity was not damaged, but could not work properly for a while because of swelling and bruising. Or it may have been that another bit of the brain which was needed to work with the control part was out of action for a while, for the same sort of reasons. This kind of 'recovery of function', or getting back an ability which was affected by the head injury, generally takes place in the earlier period after the accident, and it generally happens whether or not you are trying to practise that skill.

Sometimes recovery happens because parts of the brain which are not damaged get used to taking over some of the job of the damaged bit. How this happens we do not know exactly, but it is clear that if the brain is to find a new way to do the particular activity which has been damaged, that activity has to be practised many times.

There are two important points about recovery after brain damage. The first is that how soon and how much improvement takes place is affected by the frequency and type of rehabilitation. The other important point is that there is always a limit to how much recovery can take place. This limit is set by the kind of injury, the amount of damage, and the age and lifestyle of the head-injured person.

THE TWO-YEAR MYTH

Many older textbooks make a very clear but quite incorrect statement about recovery after a head injury. They say that all the recovery that can be expected will take place in the first two years after the accident. This is simply not true. Not only is it not true, but it has caused much needless stress and unhappiness in families and patients who were given this incorrect information. You do not need to retire to bed on the eve of the second anniversary of the accident, believing that if your relative or friend is not walking yet, for example, then he is doomed to spend the rest of his life in a wheelchair. This may indeed be so, but two years is much too soon after the injury to give up hope, and to give up trying.

> **People have continued to improve five, ten, or more years after a head injury**

It is correct that the time when the most recovery takes place is in the first six months after the injury. This is partly because of the mechanism we described earlier where parts of the brain cannot work properly in the early stages because of bruising and swelling around them. But because improvement takes place at a slower rate in the next six months does not mean that it will eventually slow to zero.

If you are given the two-year myth, ask your doctor to confirm what we have told you. You might also like to ask around at the next Head-Injury Support Group which you attend. You will find no shortage of people to tell you about the progress which their relatives made well beyond the two-year period.

SUPPORT FOR THE CARE-GIVER

You will see from the last section that when we talk about recovery after a head injury we are talking about what can be a very long-term affair. Even if your relative or friend eventually regains his independence, he may need you as a care-giver for many months. You will need to support him when he feels despondent about how little progress he has made.

You will need to comfort him if his old friends neglect him, or if his brothers or sisters no longer bring their friends home to visit.

There are two things that you need to do. The first is to bring out that diary which we talked about earlier, the one you started while he was still in hospital. Read it through with him and you will be amazed at how much progress there has been since then. You will, we hope, have kept up with making a daily entry in this diary. The second thing which you need to do is to compare how the head-injured person is now with how he was two or three months ago, not with how he was before the accident happened.

Chapter 10 talks about coping with the long-term adjustments which need to be made when someone in the family has had a severe head-injury, and will never make a full recovery. Use some of that advice to get you through the stage when you are helping your relative or friend on the road to an independent life. We have already given you the most important advice, however, which is to look forwards and not back. Make the comparison between how he is now and how he was a few months ago, and set some realistic goals about how you would like him to be in a few months time again.

Finally, you need to realize that you will not be able to help anyone if you make yourself ill looking after him. Allow yourself to have days off. Even if you do not have any relatives or friends who can mind the patient for you, the social worker at the hospital, or else your Head-Injury Society Support Group, will arrange someone to sit with him. Do not be shy about asking for this help. Further on down the track you will be able to do the same thing for another family, and you will find out just how rewarding it is to give another carer a break.

CASE HISTORIES

Michael:

Some time after the failure of the magic memory cure, Michael's parents requested an interview with his consultant. They explained that they were worried that he was taking so long to recover, that he was improving so slowly, and they wanted to know the answer to a question which they had dreaded asking before. The question was 'would Michael ever be able to go back to his university studies?' The consultant spent time going over how much progress Michael had made, and also pointed out that following a head injury, less than a year after the accident was still very early days. The consultant did not answer the question, but he did arrange for Michael to be seen by a guidance counsellor who was used to working with head-injured patients, and who would, in co-operation with the rehabilitation team, try to sort out a programme that Michael would be able to cope with.

When they met with the team again, after this consultation, Michael and his parents were a little disappointed to hear that it would be unrealistic for Michael to carry on with the law course which he had started. However, they accepted the counsellor's suggestion that Michael should change to a course which would use his good mathematical ability. They also realized that although Michael's memory problem was a disability, it did not need to prevent him from completing a university degree, as would have been the case if he had lost the ability to comprehend or to reason.

Mary:

Although Mary's behaviour had improved since the time at the special school, there had not been much change in how quickly she did things, and Mary's mother was pleased to have the volunteer help to get Mary ready. There was no longer any problem about the job since Mary's mother had this help, but she still had to make do with less sleep, and she did not have much time to spend with her husband or the other children.

It was obvious to the volunteer helper that relations between Mary's mother and father were not good. The volunteer realized that Mary's parents needed some help, and she was comfortable enough with them both to suggest that they meet with other parents who had had the same problems. Although Mary's parents had been given the information about the local support group for families of head-injured patients, neither had had the time or the energy to attend. The helper organized a baby-sitter for Mary and her sisters, and persuaded the parents to come along with her to a meeting.

Mary's mother found it helpful to talk to other mothers. Mary's father found it depressing. From the time of the accident Mary's father had taken a back seat, doing what he could to help, but waiting for the time when Mary would be better and things would get back to normal. At the support-group meeting Mary's father met parents of children who had been injured five or ten years before and who were still looking after their sons or daughers. While Mary's mother focused on the advice that every head injury was different, and that Mary's recovery would take place at Mary's own pace and in her own time, Mary's father focused on the number of years after an accident that other people had had to continue caring for a head-injured child. After this meeting he became quieter and withdrew even more from the family.

The support groups became a source of help for Mary's mother, and she came to look forward to the evenings when they were held. She found that because of her training other mothers accepted her advice, and she found it satisfying when something which she had suggested helped another family cope. However, this involvement became another barrier between Mary's mother and her husband, who began to resent the fact that she was prepared to spend the little spare time which she had with strangers and not with him.

Arnold:

During their holiday, there were many times when Arnold and his lady friend were able to forget that he had ever had an accident. There were some things which he could not cope with, such as the hotel disco with its flashing lights and loud music, but while they were swimming, relaxing, or lying in the sun he managed in his old way.

Arnold even managed for a while after the holiday ended and they returned home. This was because he was still in what he called the 'holiday-mode'. Arnold had no business to worry about now, and no need to keep to a rigid timetable. His lady friend, however, could not take an indefinite holiday from her own career, and as time went by she became increasingly irritated by his *laissez-faire* attitude. She could not understand how Arnold could cope with the holiday, but yet not have the energy to mow the lawn, let alone think about earning a living. She began to believe that Arnold was indeed a has-been, and began to treat him as one. Not surprisingly, the relationship ended for the second time.

9. Back to work and study

For months everyone involved in the head-injured victims' rehabilitation has been working towards getting him fit enough to go back to work, school, or college. Unfortunately return to work is sometimes botched, in spite of the very best of intentions. There are several ways in which this can happen. The victim can be returned to work or school before he has recovered sufficiently to cope with it, often because neither the family nor the employer or school-teacher want to hurt his feelings by telling him that it is too early. He can be returned to an inappropriate work or school environment because there has not been sufficient communication between the rehabilitation team, the employer or school, and the victim and the family. Finally, things can go very wrong if there is no system for monitoring the success of the return to work or school trial. By looking at the ways in which return to work or school can go wrong, we can arrive at some general principles which we can use to set up a better system. Remember, however, that in this section we are talking about returning the head-injured person to the employment or study which he was doing at the time of the accident. This is not always possible.

After the description of an ideal 'back to work or school' system we discuss ways of finding an employment or educational slot that the victim can cope with if the old slot is no longer the right one. The last part of the chapter talks about people with special employment problems; executives, the self-employed, the unemployed, the school dux, and the school dunce. Firstly, however, there are three basic questions about getting back into the real world.

Managing the return to work or school

Ensure that:
the head-injured person is well enough to go back
the head-injured person can cope with the environment
there is a system of monitoring the trial back at work or school

WHEN IS THE VICTIM READY TO GO BACK TO WORK?

There are quite clearly defined standards which head-injured people need to meet before they can be considered fit to work. The first is that attention and concentration span must be sufficient to allow him to work effectively and safely for a specified portion of the work day. The second is that he has maintained or regained the special skills that the job needs. The third is that he has the social skills which means that his return to work will not disrupt the routine of the work-place.

Before going back to work after a head injury

Attention and concentration must be adequate
The special skills required by the job must be adequate
Social skills must be adequate

From the time that the head-injured victim wakes up after the accident and moves into the care of the rehabilitation team, the specialists will have been monitoring his ability to attend or concentrate, they will have been monitoring his ability to cope with the demands of the job or education, and they will have been monitoring his social skills. For this reason, the members of the rehabilitation team have all the information which is needed to answer the question about when return to work or study should begin. Problems arise if this advice is ignored.

Telling the victim that he has not yet recovered sufficiently well to cope with work may not necessarily be enough to convince him that he is not yet ready. In Chapter 5 we explained how in the early stages after injury people often lack insight, and do not have the ability to judge how well they are doing. While he still has poor insight he will not be able to understand why he is being kept away from work, because it can seem to him that he does not have any problems. Sometimes even although he is aware that memory is not as good as it used to be, or that he finds it difficult to concentrate, he may not appreciate that the way he copes with these problems makes it difficult for the other people at work or school. If he has to ask a question or pass on some information as soon as he thinks of it (because otherwise he will forget it), for example, or if he needs to get up and walk around or do something different when he cannot concentrate, employers or school teachers will not be impressed by the disruption which this causes.

If the victim insists that he is right about fitness to work and that the rehabilitation team is wrong then it can be very difficult for the family. Even if the family have doubts themselves about whether or not the head-injured person will be able to cope, it can seem as if they are 'ganging up' against him if they try to persuade him to wait a while longer. It can also be difficult to resist the temptation to believe that perhaps he might be right after all. This is especially likely if families have had to listen to continual complaints that every activity which is suggested to him is boring, and that the only thing which he wants is to get back to work or to school. Although families can accept the explanation of the rehabilitation team that the 'boredom' is more likely to be frustration because the victim does not have the ability to concentrate on the activities long enough to succeed, and because he tires so quickly that anything he does quickly becomes tedious, they want him to be happy.

Sometimes family members or friends do not understand how the head injury has caused the problems. They may label the victim as lazy, unmotivated, or if they are teenagers, as 'anti-authority', 'anti-parent', or 'anti-school'. If this applies in your case, it is important that you arrange a meeting so that the relatives or friends can talk to the rehabilitation team. This will help everyone to understand why head-injured patients behave as they do, and if he is adolescent, which problems are to do with the injury and which are to do with growing up.

The situation becomes even more difficult if the employer or teacher also succumbs to the desire of the head-injured person to return to work or to school. In the typical scenario some time after the victim has left hospital he calls to visit his employer. The employer may be unaware of the typical after-effects of head injury, or may not notice much change during the space of a short visit. If there are no obvious physical signs that he has not made a full recovery the employer is very likely either to ask when the victim is coming back to work, or to agree to the suggestion that he starts back soon. On the other hand, where it is very obvious to the employer that the victim is still impaired as a result of the accident, a misguided sense of compassion may lead him or her to offer to have the victim back at work whenever he wants, and a promise that there will be something suitable for him to do.

In some cases the only practical way of managing is to allow him to have his way, and to find out for himself. If he does go back to work too soon after a significant head injury he will soon find that the tiredness this brings on makes his other problems worse. He may complain of more frequent headaches, he may have more problems remembering things, and he may lose control of temper more often. The harder he tries, the worse it may be. The tired, head-injured victim makes more mistakes, forgets more messages, makes poorer decisions, and becomes more and more frustrated with the lack of progress which goes hand in hand with this sort of tiredness. If these problems are allowed to develop they can cause friction with other employees or with the employer. At best there may be a loss of job satisfaction, while at worst things may deteriorate and lead to demotion, redundancy, resignation, or dismissal.

Sometimes the decision about return to work is made without all the information from the rehabilitation team being used. This happens particularly when the family and employer are so impressed by the physical recovery that the head-injured patient has made that they assume that there has been equivalent recovery in cognitive function. It also happens when the accident has caused multiple injuries, and there are several different specialists involved. There may be a breakdown in communication between the different disciplines working with your relative or friend and the orthopaedic specialist, for example, may clear the victim as fit for work without being aware that he still has not recovered sufficiently from the head injury to cope. Unfortunately there is also sometimes a breakdown in communication between the rehabilitation team and the family doctor. General practitioners cannot be expected to make an informed decision about return to work if they have not been kept informed of the progress of their patient, but they are the health professionals that the patient knows best, and they are most likely to be approached about getting back to work.

WHAT WORK SHOULD THE PATIENT GO BACK TO?

To the victim, there is only one answer to this question, and that is to go back to the work that he was doing before the accident. Usually, however, there needs to be some compromise when he first goes back. This is because normally he will be starting work before he has made a complete recovery. In Chapter 5 we described some of the continuing effects of the injury. These effects put some constraints on how much he can do.

First, because he is likely to tire quickly, the victim will be unable to last out a full day when he starts back to work, and so the job has to be part time. Related to this is how well he has regained control of the emotional system, because he will be more likely to lose control of his temper if he is over-tired. The rehabilitation team may suggest that the victim should be given jobs where he does not have to deal with the public if this is likely to put him under pressure.

Next, because he will not be able to concentrate as well as he used to, the job needs to be structured to take into account his ability to concentrate. He will cope better if he does not have to work in noisy surroundings, for example, or where there is a lot to distract him. Because reaction times are likely to be slower than normal, he may not be safe using machinery, or driving a vehicle. If memory is not yet working well he needs to be given jobs where there will not be too many demands on memory, or where he can compensate by using memory aids. He will often have problems with balance, and so may need to avoid those parts of the job where he would need to work from ladders or scaffolding. Finally, as well as the head injury there are often other injuries which limit what work can be done.

In most cases one member of the team (usually the occupational therapist) will need to visit the work-place to check that the victim will be able to manage.

HOW DO WE KNOW WHETHER OR NOT THE WORK TRIAL IS SUCCEEDING?

For most people the first few days at a new job or at a new school are very exciting. The excitement is great also for people who have had to take time off work because of a head injury. When the victim is eventually cleared to return to work the excess adrenaline will probably carry him through the first week. For this reason, we need to look at how he is doing three or four weeks after he gets back, not how he did on the first three or four days.

The four parties who have a primary interest in the 'return-to-work' situation are the head-injured person, the employer, the rehabilitation team, and the care-giver. All these people should be involved in the evaluation of the work trial. The team will usually set up a system for getting a weekly report from the employer, and they will modify the work hours depending on that report. Sometimes this does not happen, and the unfortunate head-injured person is stuck in a work trial which is too limited or too demanding for much longer than necessary because of this lack of supervision.

Sometimes the employer does not want to change the system, because as long as he or she has the victim on a work trial wages do not have to be paid. The employer has no incentive to approach the rehabilitation team, the insurers, or the head-injured person to point out to them that the work trial does have an economic potential. In such a case an independent assessment of the work may be needed.

Although the victim is the central character in the return-to-work arrangements, because of the head injury he is usually the least able to judge how he is doing. The basis of the problem of lack of insight was discussed in Chapter 5. Because of this the contribution from families or care-givers is very important. They will know if the victim is over-tired when he gets home, or if he is becoming more irritable, restless, or aggressive at home. These are very clear signs that the hours of work should be cut back, and the rehabilitation team must be informed. The victim may see this as a retrograde step, but the desire to spare his feelings should not stop the care-givers from doing this. The team members will explain that reducing the hours of a work trial does not mean that it was a failure. On the contrary, it is a sign of a successful trial where there is good communication between the people who are monitoring progress.

A SYSTEM FOR RETURNING TO PRE-INJURY EMPLOYMENT OR STUDY

Planning

Planning for return to work or school will start before the victim has reached the stage where the trial can begin. By the time that he is well enough to go back someone from the rehabilitation team will have visited the employer or teacher and will have explained the sorts of problems that the head injury has caused. Together they will have worked out what parts of the job he will be able to manage, and what changes will need to be made for him. If he normally works on a noisy factory floor, for example, he may need to start back in another area, say in the stockroom. Because it will be hard for the head-injured child to cope with the noise and bustle of a normal classroom, the school needs to arrange some quiet periods where he can have time out. Ideally, arrangements should be made for him to work with a tutor to catch up on work that has been missed.

It will have been explained to the employer or the teacher that the victim will not be able to cope with a full day at work or school. It will also have been explained that he is likely to have some days where he may not be able to cope as well, or for as long, as he does on other days. Arrangements will have been made for him to have a place to lie down if he is unwell with headache, or to leave early if necessary.

Starting small

When the victim has made enough recovery to start back at work or school, a meeting will be set up with all the people involved; the head-injured person, the care-givers, the employer or teacher, and the rehabilitation team. The reason for this meeting is so that everyone is clear about the plans, and to arrange for systems to check how the trial is doing. Although it may seem to the victim and the family that the trial is too restricted, the team members will explain that it is important to 'start small'. The team will stress that it is better to err on the side of caution when the hours of the trial are set. Two or three hours a day for two or three days a week are usually enough to start with, and these will be morning hours when he is most alert. The time will be built up only when it is clear that he can cope at home as well as at work.

Checking

Usually the rehabilitation team will continue to see the victim on the days that he is not at work or school to monitor how he is doing. There will also be regular reviews of the hours, and regular contact with the employer or school teacher to make sure that any unexpected problems are dealt with. We have already explained the important part that the care-giver plays during this stage, in providing information on how well the victim can cope when he is at home. A good return-to-work system will include families and care-givers in the review meetings.

Sometimes the only change that needs to be made in work conditions is in the hours of work, because fatigue is such a limiting factor. Where part-time work or part-time attendance at school is something which has to be accepted as a long-term condition, it is important to remember that supervisors and school-teachers will eventually change. The new people cannot be expected to know why the hours are restricted, or to understand the problems which the head-injured person has. It is important to make sure that if there is to be a change in personnel someone will be responsible for passing on information to the new person.

ALTERNATIVE EMPLOYMENT

We have already pointed out how people who tire more quickly and more deeply after head injury are limited in the number of hours that they can spend doing effective work. This problem also applies to the many cases who have not been able to go back to their old job, even on a part-time basis. However, before they get to this stage, they have already faced the problem of what work should they do instead? There are several obvious constraints. For example, if he has an arm or a leg that does not work very well the head-injured person cannot do a physically demanding job. If there are problems with thinking quickly or with remembering he will not be able to cope with a high-pressure job.

Once the victim has accepted that he needs to change what he does for a living, he may be tempted to select a new occupation which is attractive but unrealistic. If he is advised that he will have to find a desk job, for example, he may opt for being an accountant when his aptitude is more suited to that of a clerk. We have already explained in Chapter 5 how head injury affects the ability to make complex decisions, and the victim is usually not able on his own to judge which new occupation suits him best. Obviously his likes and dislikes need to be taken into account, but he also needs help from the family and from the rehabilitation team who will be able to judge whether or not he has the ability to re-train for a particular job.

Sometimes it is not only the unrealistic judgement of the victim which guides the choice of an inappropriate new career. If he and the family have always been high-achievers, it is difficult for them all to accept that the victim must move to a less demanding job, or one which they see as of lower status. Unfortunately it is a fact that many people are left with permanent problems after a head injury that limit what job they can do. Families and care-givers need to realize that it is much kinder to their relative or friend to guide him to a job which he will be able to cope with, rather than to allow him to take on something in which he has no possibility of succeeding.

SOME GROUPS WITH SPECIAL PROBLEMS

Executives and managers

People in demanding and high-powered occupations have special difficulty getting back to work because the effect of head injury is to impair the skills which they need most. Decision making and ability to concentrate need to have recovered to a better level than for someone who has to return to a routine or repetitive job. So executives will have a longer period after injury before they can get back to work at all. Even the most secure person will be concerned about his position, and about what changes may have been made in his absence.

Executives and managers need special guidance to help them return to the work-force, but they are understandably reluctant to have their employers and associates learn about the accident or the problems which it has caused. For this reason the victim needs an experienced and authoritative counsellor who can help him rearrange his work schedule so that he will be able to cope. The most demanding meetings or appointments must be made for early in the day, for example, and he needs to use his authority to defer important decisions until he has had enough time to consider them. He also needs to accept and use any devices such as tape recorders which will take some of the load off his memory.

Finally, many people in this category are no longer young. In Chapter 7 we described how older people may not ever make a complete recovery. The possibility that the victim may need to change to a less demanding job or to take early retirement needs to be faced.

The self-employed

Even when a person who is self-employed has adequate accident insurance it is often difficult for him to stay away from work for as long as he should. If the business is small there may not be anyone else with the skill which is needed to keep it going. If it is a larger concern he may worry about supervising the staff. If he has little or no insurance, financial difficulties may force him to try to cope at work before he is well enough to do this. In addition, he has the same problems as outlined in the last section for the executive.

Sometimes it may be possible for him to employ someone to take his place. Sometimes a better alternative may be to consider selling the business before it runs down because of his absence. Where possible, a business associate or friend should be brought in to help the head-injured victim and the family reach the most sensible decision.

The unemployed

Although it may seem strange to talk about return to work for someone who does not have any work to return to, the unemployed person has special problems after he has had a head injury. This is because starting a work trial is an important stage of the rehabilitation process, and it is always more successful if it can be done in familiar surroundings at the place where the victim was employed before the accident. If he has few or no work skills it may be difficult to find a place for him. If, as is often the case, he receives no accident insurance he may not be able to manage financially unless he finds paid work.

There are several problems in finding paid employment. Because of the head injury the victim will be less likely to cope well with a job interview. He may not be able to answer questions quickly, or may not have regained social skills and the ability to judge how he is presenting. In addition, most employers prefer to take on someone who has not been off work for any length of time. When part of the period of unemployment is because of a head injury, the head-injured victim is often even less acceptable as an employee.

The above-average student

Ability to learn and to concentrate is impaired after even minor head injuries. No matter how bright the student is this will affect his ability to cope with school. Although he has the advantage of an above average store of knowledge, in most cases he has the disadvantage of never having had to work hard at his studies. He has not had to go over and over something that he wishes to learn in order to remember it later, and it can be shattering for him to find that this is what he now needs to do. Compared to others in the class, he may now learn things as quickly as expected. Compared to how he was before, the memory problem is very obvious.

Similar situations arise with other effects of the injury. Because he starts out with above-average ability, he may be able to cope with things at a good average level yet still be genuinely impaired by the accident. Where the problem is a severe one, so that he cannot even cope at an average level, a good student will need extra counselling. This is not just to help him to cope with the loss, but to help him re-direct his curricula so that he can make the best use of intact abilities.

The below-average student

Poor students also have special problems after a head injury. Because he has had poor academic records, it can be easy for families and teachers to miss that he has a genuine memory or language problem as a result of the head injury. If he was already 'learning-disabled', he will need to have a very severe memory problem before this is obvious in school performance. If he was a poor reader then the effect of damage to the parts of the brain that affect skills like reading will be less obvious.

Because the child has not done well at school, he will have less established learning to build on and to help compensate for these problems. He may also have lost the ability to take part in the non-academic school activities, such as sports, where the learning disability was not a handicap. Again counselling is important to help the child understand why things are even harder for him and to guide him with alternate activities which he may be able to cope with.

CASE HISTORIES

Michael:

Exactly 18 months after his accident Michael attended the first lecture of the 'Introduction to computer' course which he had enrolled in at his old university. Many people had been involved in the arrangements for him to do this. Michael and his parents had spent ages looking at courses which he could cope with, and they had come up with this one, which was designed mainly for students who were not prepared to commit themselves to a full degree course. The course ran for 12 months, with just two lectures a week and one laboratory session. Once they had decided on the course, the counsellor from the rehabilitation team had talked with all the faculty members who would be involved with Michael, so that they all knew the problems which Michael had with memory and concentration. The social worker had arranged for Michael to stay in a university hostel for the first six months, so that he would not have to cope with his own flat and looking after himself as well as with lectures. The rehabilitation officer had arranged for Michael to have a portable cassette recorder so that he did not have to worry about taking notes during the lectures.

Michael felt a little ambivalent about having all this extra help, but he was so keen to return to university that he accepted it anyway. Michael's father was a little disappointed that his son was not doing a proper degree course, but he managed to keep this disappointment from Michael. Michael's mother was pleased that her son was so happy about the move, but she also felt a little guilty that part of her pleasure was in regaining some of the independence which she had given up ever since Michael had his accident.

The rehabilitation team were also pleased. Although they would be monitoring how Michael managed at the university, and would not discharge him from their care until they were sure that he could cope, each team member was satisfied with the part that he or she had played in bringing Michael through to this stage.

Mary:

Mary went back to school the week her father left the family. The social worker thought that it would be best for Mary to be away from the house, and Mary's mother was too shocked by the break-up of her marriage to demur. Because the move back to school was precipitated by the family crisis, the usual groundwork to prepare the teachers and the other pupils had not been done. It was not quite two years since the accident.

Mary was so excited at the thought of returning to school the next day that she hardly slept. The sound of her mother weeping during the night penetrated her consciousness but it did not bother her. Her old friend, the retired school teacher, was asleep in the spare bed in Mary's room, and had come to cushion Mary from the upheaval. Mary woke her several times to check whether or not she should start to get ready.

Mary was bombarded by questions from the other children, and was the centre of attention on the first day. The headmaster made a point of welcoming her at the school assembly, and Mary was placed in the class that she would have moved to if she had not had the accident. Mary could not understand much of what the teacher was talking about, and she found it hard to sit still for a whole period. Mary's new teacher allowed her to spend the day listening and did not expect any work from her, but Mary was still very tired by lunch time. At the lunch break the other children in her class had jostled to sit next to her. Mary liked that, and liked the way that they made her laugh. Mary did not realize that this was because her laugh went on and on, which the other children thought very amazing.

When Mary went back into the classroom in the afternoon she was still laughing, and the teacher was quite cross with her. The teacher was cross also when Mary could not keep her eyes open and went to sleep on her desk. Even so, Mary was keen to go back to school the next day and she was a bit worried that the new teacher might not let her. She was so worried that she ran up to the front of the classroom to ask the teacher for reassurance. The teacher was in the middle of explaining the principles of multiplication to the class at the time and she was not pleased with the interruption.

Mary was allowed one more day in that class, but she was just as distractible and proved such a distraction to the other children that she was moved to another class. This was the class which Mary had been in when she had had the accident, and the same teacher was in charge. The teacher knew Mary well, and realized that her behaviour was not deliberate naughtiness. She also realized that the hustle and noise of a big classroom made it even harder for Mary to cope. By rearranging the timetable and calling on Mary's old friend to help, the teacher was able to organize Mary's day so that sessions in the classroom were alternated with rests, and with time in a quiet room having lessons on her own under the supervision of her old friend. This worked much better. The other children in the class did not remember Mary from the year before, and so did not expect her to behave in any particular way with them. During classroom time the teacher was able to make sure that Mary was not singled out as odd or different, and that she could cope with the activities that she was given.

By the end of the year Mary had made some gains at school, and the issue of the move to another class had to be faced. Mary's mother wanted her to be moved into the class with others of her own age. Fortunately, this was not done. Mary's teacher was very aware that Mary spent most of her time in the playground with children younger than she was, and that most of Mary's old friends had become rather unkind and teased her unmercifully. The teacher realized that not only would Mary find it hard to cope with the work in the higher class, but that she would be unhappy in the company of her former friends. So Mary continued her education a year behind her peers. With the help of a sensible teacher who was sensitive to her needs, she was able to remain in the normal school system. Eventually even Mary's mother accepted that this was a considerable achievement.

Arnold:

Two years after his accident, Arnold was still not well enough to earn a living. Because of the attitude of some of his former friends, who tended to make comments such as 'But the accident was years ago, old man' when they found that he was not working, he had stopped visiting his old clubs and other places where he used to spend his leisure time. Against the advice of the rehabilitation team, Arnold decided to move to another town, but this did not work out. He did not manage to make a new set of friends, he could not get used to the new surroundings, and he missed the support which he had had from the other people in his out-patient programme.

Arnold became very depressed, and when his daughter visited him she was so concerned about him that she persuaded him to return to his old home town so that she could 'keep an eye on him'. At first Arnold was a bit ambivalent about this. He did not enjoy his new life and he wanted to go back, but did not feel comfortable about having his daughter treat him as if he was a child.

Things did get better, however. With the help of the Rehabilitation Officer Arnold found a part-time voluntary job working with learning-disabled children. His old experience as a school teacher stood him in good stead. Although Arnold was able to manage only two to three hours before he became too tired to cope, he found that he enjoyed the feeling of accomplishment that he now had at the end of the day. He also enjoyed the sense of purpose that this gave back to his life. As the years went by Arnold accepted that age was against him, and he was unlikely to ever be able to return to paid employment. However, he was able to continue working with the children until he retired, and he proved to be a valuable source of help and information to the other members of the staff.

10. Long-term adjustment

It is a sad fact that not all head-injured patients will recover well enough for return to work or school ever to be considered. Even if these people carefully follow all the advice given in the last chapter, and even if they have extremely supportive families and employers, if they do not get back the mental and physical skills which they need to function in full open employment, they will never be able to take this step.

If you have read this book through from the beginning, you will know by now that recovery from head injury can often take many years. It is also important to realize that recovery may never be complete. At some stage you and your family member or friend may need to come to terms with this, and to accept that the life which you all had before the accident is over. This is a step which you must take before you can all alter your expectations and set up some more realistic goals for yourselves.

It is very difficult to come to terms with this incomplete recovery. You may feel that you are giving up hope, and also that, in a sense, you are letting down the person who had the accident. But until you and the injured person do make adjustments, you run the risk of building up unnecessary frustration, because if your expectations of what the future will bring are unrealistic you are really setting up the victim for failure. This chapter outlines some of the steps that may help you to work through this difficult period. Note, however, that this advice cannot replace individual counselling from someone who knows your special circumstances. It is important that you talk to your family doctor about how you can get this special help.

LETTING GO

One of the most difficult things about accepting that the accident has put an end to the life which your family member or friend had is that he *is* still alive. If the worst had happened, and the patient had died, you would by now have gone through the grieving process. You would have had the opportunity to mourn the passing of the victim, with a funeral where you, your family, and friends could pay tribute to him, and you could publicly acknowledge that he had gone from you. But you cannot do that now. You can see the 'old' person every day. Even if the victim is unable to walk or communicate, he has the same shaped face, the same hair colour, and he may have some of the same mannerisms, maybe the same glint in the eye when he is being stubborn. This is certainly not a stranger who has taken the place of the person you knew and loved. This 'new' character, however, has lost many of the things which made up the old life. You all need to accept these losses, and to get on with making a new life.

When should you make this decision? We have already said that it may seem that you are giving up. You may also feel that if you do not keep pushing, and your friend or family member stops trying, then he will not have any chance to recover. But we are not advising that you and he sit back and say, 'Well, this is it. This is how it is always going to be.' What 'letting go' means is that you need to let go of the things from the life before the accident that are impossible for the victim now. The ideal time for this to take place is as soon as you are able to come to terms with the fact that there have been these losses. Later on we shall discuss how you can help the victim to let go too, but for now we will concentrate on you, the person who is the care-giver.

Your relative or friend may have been keen on sports but may have had no interests outside the sport of his choice. However, no amount of will-power will allow him to run a marathon with paralysed legs, or if he is still uncoordinated and has poor balance. Having 'running in the marathon' as the goal is unrealistic at either stage. It will also hinder him from looking around for other activities or interests which could be practical and possible for him to do now. You and he need to let go the person who was a budding marathon champion, and work at a level which is appropriate now for someone with his handicaps. This advice applies equally to the law student who cannot speak clearly, to the apprentice who has lost the ability to control his hands, or to the artist who has lost his sight. You need to let go the person who had the potential to follow these careers.

We have already talked about the way head injury affects mood and temperament. We have explained how fatigue can be a persistent problem, and how the sleep cycle can be disturbed. We have also explained how making decisions can be more difficult, and how the victim may no longer be able to appreciate the effect on others of what he does and says. All these things make up 'personality', and it is not surprising that families often talk about how the injury has changed the victim's personality. In the sense that personality can be defined by the sum of the ways that we react to the things which happen to us, then if he reacts differently to the way he would have done before the accident, your relative or friend does have a different personality now. But this does not mean that he is a different person. Although it may be hard to do, you will find that you cope much better with the effects of the accident once you can let go of the pre-injury personality, and accept that your partner or relative or friend now reacts in a different way.

All this is easier for you to accept than it is for the person who has had the head injury. We all have a picture of ourselves and the sort of person that we are. Psychologists call this our self-image. We suspect that it takes a long time for the self-image to change after a head injury. Even if he needs to use wheelchairs to get around, for example, and has problems making other people understand what he says, or reacts irrationally at times, a head-injured person will resent being placed in a facility for physically handicapped or psychiatric patients because he does not see himself as disabled. Neither does he have anything in common with the other patients. For a long time people who have had a head injury still consider themselves to be young, healthy, and able; a person who happens to have had an accident, so at the moment needs to use a wheelchair.

We need to realize that for a long time head-injury victims still think of themselves as they were before their accidents

---

It is important for you and his friends and relatives to remember that this is how the victim sees himself. To him, he is as physically attractive, as witty, and the same good company as he was before his injury. Unhappily, it is obvious to those around him that he is not, and people naturally respond very differently to the 'new' person that he has become. Indeed, very often embarrassing or unacceptable behaviour can be interpreted by those around him as a desperate attempt on his part to prove that he is the same old self, because of the way others now respond to him.

We said earlier that we would talk about ways to help your relative or friend come to terms with the fact that the accident has changed him, and that he needs to change what he expects to get out of life. In essence this means that we need to get him to face up to the fact that the self-image which he carries from the days before the accident is no longer accurate. This does not mean that you get him to replace it with the negatives of 'failure, crippled, ugly, or useless'. It is for this very reason that you, the rehabilitation staff, and the counsellors will have tried to find something that he can succeed at to replace the things that he can no longer do. This is simply what is meant by the advice to set realistic goals. You need to help him feel good about himself because of the things that he can do, not bad because of the things that he cannot do. We cannot stress too strongly that you need to make sure that he has appropriately trained counsellors to help him through this.

You, as the non head-injured person in your relationship, will need to work out the changes that your family member or friend will have to make, as well as the changes which you must make yourself. You may also have to act as a back-up counsellor for him. Again, this is a difficult role, especially if he is a parent or partner. It is worth repeating the advice that we gave earlier; that is, do not be too proud to ask relatives and friends for their help and support.

Eventually you will reach the stage where you are ready to accept the fact that the accident has changed what you can expect from your loved one. There are many different emotions that you will feel on the way to this acceptance. Before we talk about ways in which you can handle some of these emotions, it is important to remember that these are perfectly natural reactions to the losses which you have had. It is at this stage that you and your family most need support from your local head-injury group, and reassurance that there are other people who have been through the same process.

GRIEF

We have already pointed out that when a victim does not survive a head injury, family and friends are able to grieve for him, and eventually to move on to life without him. It is important to remember that you need to grieve also for the things which the accident has taken away from you, even though you have not physically lost him. It is normal and natural to be sad that your relative or friend is so different from the way he was before the injury. It is normal and natural to be sad that he can no longer be the companion who was able to share the interests which you had. It is normal and natural to be sad that you have lost the support of your partner or parent.

You need to accept also that it is all right to cry. Probably at this stage the victim will not be ready to let go of the way he was before the accident. Neither will he be ready to grieve. But you can. You are allowed to cry for what you have lost. Do not feel guilty that this somehow implies that you are crying because he survived, and that you wish that he had died rather than be left with such handicaps. Do not feel guilty that you are being self-indulgent and should be able to 'keep a stiff upper lip'. Crying can be a very good safety valve.

Work through your grief

Allow yourself to cry
Allow yourself to remember the past
Allow others to talk about the past
Accept that the past is behind you
Accept that the future will be different

When you get to this stage you need to allow yourself some time alone when you can weep for what has gone, and when you have the opportunity re-live, through photographs and mementoes, how things were before the accident. Some people find that it also helps to make a list of the things which have been lost, or to put together in one album a record of your friend or relative's sporting or academic achievements. The important thing to realize is that the list and the album are from the past, that they are from the different life that you had before the accident.

You also need to encourage his friends to talk to you about the things which your relative or friend used to say and do. Finally, encourage other members of the family to talk about the things which you all did together, and that the victim will not be able to do again. It is not morbid to appreciate the past and to mourn for it. It may be that having a good cry together will help you all.

ANGER

Anger is a common and natural response following a head injury. We are all familiar with this 'why me?' type of anger. Many of the losses which a head injury brings about are very hard to accept and anger can be an issue for your friend or relative throughout his rehabilitation.

Most often the anger is expressed against close relatives and friends, not because they deserve it, but because they are most trusted. By this we mean that it is safe for him to be himself when he is with people he

relies on for support. When he is away from home he may be able to
make the extra effort and hide his anger from acquaintances or employers.
If he showed this anger too often with them it might lead to rejection or
loss of employment. For relatives and care-givers this can be hurtful, and
they need to understand that this does not mean lack of respect or love
on his part.

In our experience the 'anger phase' is just that—a phase which will
generally pass. In the meantime if anger is a problem in your family here
are a few suggestions that may help. If the anger is so strongly expressed
that it spills over, or risks spilling over into actual hurt to others then
seek professional help. Try not to read motives into every angry out-
burst. There is often no real intent behind the anger, no plan or scheme.
He may not seem like the person you knew before the accident but it is
too early to think in terms of 'changed personality'. Personality changes,
though they can occur, are much less frequent than you might suppose.
Try to think of the anger as temporary and separate from the person you
know and love.

Ask yourself if you are being too helpful, for this can sometimes be a
trigger for his frustration. It is easy to get stuck in the groove of helping
and guiding and taking responsibility away from him. Though this may
be necessary in the early stages of recovery it can be irritating for him
later on as he tries to regain control over his life and wishes to make his
own choices. Avoid arguments, but discuss important differences when
both you and he are fresh and calm. Remember that it often makes no
sense to him either that he finds trivial things so irritating. Finally, as we
pointed out earlier, anger is often simply the result of fatigue.

Dealing with anger

The anger phase won't last.
Don't pursue arguments.
Think of the anger as separate.
Don't take the hurt to heart.
Find a safe outlet for anger (e.g. physical activity and exercise)

Your friend or relative will also experiment with different ways of coping
with anger and frustration. Physical activity and exercise is helpful to
many people, as is 'getting away from it all' for a quiet period. Others
have found some benefit from relaxation techniques. There are no easy
solutions and things which work for other people may not work for the
person with a head injury. The problem is usually one of unpredictable
flashes of anger rather than an attitude problem.

GUILT

What parent or partner of a head-injured person has not spent time agonizing over casual remarks and complaints made ages in the past, which taken out of context suggest that the victim was a nuisance and that a head injury is the least that they deserve? This reaction may occur partly because of the very human need to find an explanation for the dreadful thing that has happened. There has to be a reason why he was the one struck by a bus, and why you are being punished. It is the rare relationship where there was never any resentment on one side or the other, however momentarily, at some time in the past.

It is hard to forgive yourself for these remarks, but you need to leave your guilt outside the door and bring your normal rational mind into play. How many times have you snapped at the victim, or carped, or unfairly accused him of something? Was the victim punished with a head injury each time? Of course he was not. Why, when most of your thoughts about your partner or family member have been positive, would the one instance when you lost your temper have resulted in him being 'struck down' like this. Further, what sort of mechanism would need to be involved if every negative complaint about a person resulted in a head injury?

Sometimes assuming guilt allows us to cope with awful things like the effects of a head injury, and to find a 'reason' why it has happened. The problem is that this interferes with your relationship with your loved one. If you accept that you are to blame for their condition, then you are going to treat the victim in a different way to normal, and so you have doubly lost him. He is also likely to react differently to you if you treat him as someone that you have damaged. Again this may reinforce your sense of guilt.

Many people feel responsible for the injury because indirectly the victim was in a position to be hurt because of something that they did or did not do. Maybe the motor cycle that a son crashed on was a birthday present from his parents. Maybe the son was able to buy the hang-glider that he rode into a cliff only because his parents lent him the money. Maybe a husband was driving his car that night because his wife had asked him to collect their daughter from the school social.

Guilt is very much an emotional response. Common sense tells us that we are only responsible for the head injuries of those we have run down in cars, struck down with blunt weapons, or where we have in other ways directly inflicted the damage. Some few of us may be responsible for the injuries of the victim. For the others it is important to accept the principle of cause and effect, and to accept that no amount of taking the blame on yourself is going to alter what has happened already. The only sure consequence of acting the guilty party is that you will be a less effective care-giver.

BLAME

We have talked about the problems of taking on the responsibility yourself for the injuries that your family member has suffered. It is even more important to refrain from unfairly putting the blame on somebody else. The only advantage of having someone to blame is that it somehow 'makes sense' of what has happened. However, the price that you pay for this is out of all proportion. In most cases the person who is unfairly blamed is a family member or friend. Every one of the victim's associates is affected by the injury, and he or she needs the support of every one during the recovery stage. If one parent blames the other for letting their son borrow the family car, and therefore for the accident, their relationship will be strained and their ability to support their son compromised. If the parents blame their son's wife for encouraging his interest in polo, and therefore for the accident, it will be the victim who is damaged by the family rift. If the family blame the friend who let their son have a spin on his new motor cycle, and hold him responsible for the accident, they will not only reinforce his own guilt, but it will make it impossible for the friend to offer the support which he would like to give.

But there are many cases where responsibility for the accident is very clear. What about the careless driver who rounded a corner on the wrong side of the road? What about the drunk who drove through a red light? What about the fairground operator who sold rides on dangerous equipment? What about the construction company which did not make sure that building materials would not fall on passers by? Obviously they are all responsible for the accidents which followed, and there are two stages which your need to find someone to blame will pass through.

The first stage is retribution. The guilty party must be caught and punished. Taken to the extreme, this can be quite destructive. You can be so obsessed by the knowledge that the guilty party has not yet been found or arrested that you neglect the needs of the victim and of the other members of your family. Even after the police have at last found him or her, although this gives you tremendous satisfaction, you cannot relax. Waiting for the court case and the sentence gives you the opportunity to let your imagination run riot. You know what you would do if it was up to you; you are obsessed by the need to punish, and your every interaction with the victim feeds this obsession.

> There is no punishment that can be given to someone who has caused a head injury that will alter the way that injury has affected the victim.

The second stage is healthier. Here you want to make sure that the culprits or people like them will not be able to hurt others in the same way that they have hurt your head-injured victim. Depending on your personality, you may become an activist or a joiner, but you will want laws against drinking and driving, better safety standards, and so on. This stage fills a very real need, and it is important that you find an avenue for this kind of protest. Indeed, people who can identify a guilty party and a contributing set of circumstances which can be changed can cope better with being involved with someone who has had a severe head injury. It takes away the senselessness of the accident if you can see that because it happened some good will come. To some extent this gives you back the feeling of control over the destinies of you and your loved one, which the accident had shattered.

Unfortunately, having someone to blame sometimes means that people are trapped in the past, and do not move on to learning how to cope with the present or the future. Having someone to blame, having a focus for our anger, may satisfy our need to understand why the accident happened. It stops us taking on unnecessary guilt or unfairly ascribing blame to other relatives or friends. But it does not necessarily mean that we are then able to come to terms with the accident.

It is easy to slip into a blind alley, the 'if only' mode. If only I had not given him that motor cycle. If only you had not asked him to run that errand. If only that drunk or careless driver had not been on the road. If only that ferris wheel had been condemned. This kind of response to the effects of head injury in your relative or family member is as pointless as the search for guilt or blame. Eventually we have to accept that we are not able to turn the clock back. We have to accept that apportioning guilt, or accepting blame, will not change the outcome of the head injury one iota. In the same way, whether the drunken driver whose car went through a red light and hit your daughter is sent to gaol for twenty years, or fined a trivial amount, will not alter the course of her recovery. On the other hand, if you are able to accept that how you respond to the culprit's sentence can play a vital part in determining how well your daughter responds, you have made great strides towards understanding how you can help her cope with the effects of head injury. We have stressed the importance of looking forward, of making plans for the future and not mourning forever for the past. As long as you are in the 'if only' mode you will not be able to move on to this stage of looking forward.

DENIAL

One way of coping with an unpleasant fact is to deny that it exists. This is hard to do if the effects of the accident are easily seen, such as a paralysis or a persistent coma, or if the effects are very obvious, such as difficulty with speech. In these cases it is often the poor likelihood of recovery which is denied. If you deny that the victim will never be completely better, you do not have to worry about how your friend or relative will manage. Indeed, in the early stages, this coping mechanism is very important in helping you to maintain your sanity.

Eventually, however, the time will come when you have to accept the reality of the situation. It is where denial persists beyond this point that it can interfere with your ability to come to terms with what has happened, and to make the adjustments to your own life that have to be made. You need to work through your anger and guilt and the other emotions which we have talked about, but you cannot do this as long as you deny that there is cause for these emotions, because you pretend that every-thing will be all right.

Denial is also often used as a coping mechanism further on down the track, when there may have been reasonably good physical recovery but the victim continues to have memory, concentration, and behavioural problems. This is when it is tempting to refuse to accept that the recovery is not complete. A young man's parents may seize on an instance when he forgot something in the past, for example, as evidence that 'His memory has always been awful', or use excuses such as 'Well, he has never been able to concentrate' or 'He has never been interested in things like that' to explain why he has difficulty with simple tasks. It is easier for them to handle the evidence that his behaviour is inappropriate or embarrassing by seeing this as an extension of how he acted in the past. 'He always had a droll sense of humour', or 'He was never a conventional person'.

The problem is that this denial often coincides with the period, described in Chapter 5, in which the patients themselves lack insight or awareness of the problems which they have. We have explained how family and friends can help the victim through this stage by showing him where he makes mistakes, and how he can correct them. If family as well as the victim deny that there are any problems, no rehabilitation facility will be able to help him overcome the problems. Families who have been through this often comment that they had reached a point when they were sick of hospitals, therapists, and the accident. They wanted to carry on with life, to put the accident behind them and pretend that it had not happened. Later on, when it becomes too obvious to deny that everything is not back to normal, or when the victim himself becomes more realistic, the family are ready to get back into the recovery system. The need for 'time out' can sometimes be averted if counselling and support is kept up well beyond the early weeks after the injury.

We have looked at some of the emotions that families and care-givers need to work through as they progress towards setting up satisfactory programmes for their head-injured relative. There are three areas of change. The final sections in this chapter look at the changes that need to be made to the victim's family life, to his social life, and to his work life.

THE NEW FAMILY LIFE

Where the head-injured person is an adult son or daughter, the change from independence to dependence brings an equally drastic change to the parents' lifestyle. After some twenty years rearing a family, the parents have reached a time when they are probably more financially secure than they have ever been, and when they have their home to themselves for the first time since their early married days. Then the accident happens, and they eventually bring their injured son or daughter home. Once again the parents have a dependent person to care for, and they have to face the fact that the days when they had only themselves to please have gone. Parents also have to face the fact that they need to plan for a future when they may be too old or infirm to provide the care which the son or daughter may need.

Although the parents are returned to the role of care-givers, and the adult to the role of dependent child, the situation is not the same as it had been the first time round. The head-injured victim has usually spent several years as an adult earning his own living and looking after himself, and so the new family life demands adjustments on both sides. However, because the parents are the ones with the means and mobility to do things, it is often they who decide what the adjustments should be.

The head injury families who function best are those who, through trial and error, evolve a system where the needs for care and dependency are balanced by two other important needs—the need for privacy, and the need for some control over the situation. Both the cared-for and the care-givers need to have some time on their own. Where circumstances allow, this can be managed by modifying the family home so that the head-injured person has his or her own private apartment. However, even if this is not practical, privacy need not only be possible within the four walls of the bedroom. Family or volunteers can be organized to take the victim for the whole day once a week, for example, so that the parents can have time to themselves, or to entertain or visit their own friends. Similarly, the parents can arrange to be out of the house for set times so that the victim can entertain friends without them.

The other need for both parties is the need to have some control over what is happening. There may be a great deal that the head-injured victim has no control over because of the accident. If he cannot move around without assistance, for example, the times when he gets out of bed or shifts from one room to the next has to depend on when a care-giver is available to help him. However, even the most severely disabled victim should be given the opportunity to make as many decisions as are practical about his life. Depending on circumstances, these decisions may range from when he has his meals and what he has to eat to the disposal of income. Eventually the parents must accept that their dependent child needs to be given the right to decide what happens to him, and that he also needs to get back the right to make mistakes if that is how the decisions turn out.

The dependant in a head-injury family needs

Care
Privacy
Control

The care-givers in a head-injury family need

Support
Privacy
Control

We have focused on the most typical case, that in which the victim is young and single. The special problems that arise when he is a partner or parent have already been discussed in Chapter 7. How well your family is able to develop a new life after the accident depends not only on how willing you are as the care-giver to adapt to a changed role in this 'new' family. It also depends on whether or not the head-injured victim is able to modify his role and adjust to the changes that the accident has brought about.

THE NEW SOCIAL LIFE

Probably one of the saddest secondary effects of a severe head-injury is loneliness. In the first weeks after the injury there is usually no shortage of friends to visit the victim. The tragedy of the accident is very fresh, and the 'old' person still very real. Gradually, as the months go by, the situation changes. The frequency of visits drops rapidly. This may be because of communication problems. Talking with the victim may be such an effort that it becomes easier to put off this effort until another day. It may be because of the changed way in which he reacts. It can be very painful for friends to see their old companion behaving in an atypical way. It will also be because, as time goes by, the old friends will have met new people and they will have had new experiences that they cannot share with the victim. We all grow apart from acquaintances that we do not see regularly. When your life is in the outside world where you earn your living and pursue the leisure activities which interest you, it is not surprising that the only thing which you have in common with your old friend, whose life is confined to the hospital or rehabilitation centre, is life before the accident. It is not surprising, therefore, that there is less and less contact with old friends.

New friends are difficult to find. This applies not only to the severely disabled head-injury victim, but also to the person who has regained the ability to walk and to talk. The reasons are easy to understand. We have stressed the problems which he may have with tiredness, irritability, coping with noise, or with crowds. It is not surprising that he has difficulty coping with social gatherings too; thus is not surprising that invitations to social gatherings eventually dry up.

Community groups which have been organized to provide social activities for the disabled are not always the answer to the problem. We have discussed the long lag that there is before the head-injured victim sees himself as other than an able-bodied person. The denial mechanism we described earlier in the chapter is relevant here. Reactions to people with special needs will typically be of denial, and he may refuse to accept that he also has these needs. This is partly because the only common ground between the traumatically and congenitally disabled is the disability. Until the accident the trauma victim was able to participate in many activities that he can no longer cope with. Yet he will retain his interests, in for example, sport and fast cars. The interests of the congenitally disabled will, of necessity, be very different.

The traumatically and the congenitally disabled have little in common except the disability.

Community groups which provide venues for social activities especially for head-injured victims and their families seem to work better, possibly because the victim feels more comfortable among people who understand the problems which he has. However, there is the obvious disadvantage that this restricts his social life to the company of others like himself.

Some victims find friends outside this circle among two different age-groups. They may often find it easy to relate to the elderly, who also cannot keep up the fast pace of doing things that the peers of the head-injured victim expect. They may also often find company among younger children, who are usually delighted to find an adult who has the time to spend hours on end talking to them about a favourite subject.

THE NEW WORK LIFE

Although it is unlikely that the survivor of a very severe head injury will ever be able to return to full-time paid employment, he has the same need as everyone else to be productive. This need is recognized by most agencies, but it is not always met successfully. Sheltered workshops provide something to do to fill in the waking hours, but often the occupation that head-injured persons are given is not something which they find interesting, or that gives them satisfaction.

We believe that even when a victim can cope with some of the activities in a sheltered workshop, if he does not enjoy this work then it is not the appropriate place for him. In other words, the need to feel satisfied at the end of the day with what has been achieved outweighs the convention that he should receive payment for what he does. This means that the new work life does not necessarily mean paid employment. Neither should the new work life entail a nine-to-five job, as it is likely that the victim will not have the ability to concentrate for that period of time and would get too tired to do anything else if he did.

The task that he does should depend on his abilities and his interests. The next chapter looks at the type of rehabilitation service which would be provided in an ideal world. Vocational rehabilitation is an important part of that service, and we would hope that your relative or friend will have the help of a specialist in vocational rehabilitation to help him to discover what the new work in his new work life will be.

11. Providing a head-injury service

Up to now we have been talking about the effects of head injury and how the problems are dealt with. We have agreed that many of the problems are very difficult to solve. We have also suggested that the service that the authorities provide is often inadequate, both because they have not understood what is needed and because they have not given the requirements of head-injured people enough priority in their budgets.

In this chapter we will try to summarize the problems of management and suggest what a good head-injury service should provide. We will then look at the difficulties from the point of view of the people who have to provide a service, so that we can argue with them on their own terms. Lastly, we will suggest ways in which concerned people can influence the decision makers.

THE PROBLEMS OF MANAGEMENT

We will list the outstanding problems of management in the order in which most people meet them as the victim goes through the stages from the accident and emergency room onwards.

1. Information and relations with staff. Families and close friends need to know what is happening and to be able to ask the questions about the issues that are important to them. This runs through the whole time span.
Action: There must be a charter for management at all stages which insists on regular opportunities as of right for the family to be told what is happening and for the family to ask questions.

2. Support and understanding. Like the previous section, but looking at the more personal side of relationships. In the first stages members of the family need counselling and support in their grief and loss. Later, the victim and the family need to understand the problems which each of them has, as far as they can, and to make allowances for each other. This is needed for those with mild injuries with persisting problems as well as for those with severe injuries.

Action: Three sources of help can be used. Firstly, professional counselling must be available in the early stages of grief and loss. It may not be appreciated then, and it should be offered again as often as it seems needed. Secondly, support from family who have gone through the same problems themselves is usually welcomed later. Lastly, those who have themselves been injured and have recovered can often explain the situation better than anyone. The first counselling needs to be organized by the hospital. Later counselling may be provided through voluntary effort, by the head-injury societies, but professional guidance and monitoring should be available.

3. Hospital services in the acute stages. Most hospitals accept the need for a special trauma service, and try to organize as good a one as their situation allows. Small country hospitals have special problems, and most rely on regional services and use skilled transport teams to get patients to expert centres. When the life-threatening stage is over, around the fourth to the twelfth week after the accident, the situation is much less satisfactory. Many hospitals retain such patients in an acute-treatment setting which is not geared to their rehabilitation needs.

Action: Hospitals need to provide accommodation for patients whose primary need is rehabilitation but who still require some medical and nursing care and who are not fit to leave hospital.

Management needs—first stage

A trauma service expert in managing head injury
Information and support, as of right, whenever needed

---

4. Rehabilitation services on discharge from hospital. In many places these are limited. Expertise may not be available. The amount of treatment that can be given each week may be below the level at which it is effective if there are not enough staff, or if there are problems of transport to rehabilitation centres which result in short hours and extra fatigue.

Action: It must be possible for rehabilitation to occupy the major part of the week, without unnecessary fatigue. If it is needed, live-in accommodation must be available.

> **Management needs—second stage**
> *Expert rehabilitation services:*
> in hospital
> live-in rehabilitation
> outpatient rehabilitation

5. Return to normal occupation. It must be the aim to return every injured person to their previous occupation, or to the highest level of earning or personal satisfaction possible. Existing vocational rehabilitation organizations are often unaware of the special needs of the head-injured person or they are unable to provide the extra supervision needed.
Action: Vocational rehabilitation centres must provide staff and expertise, with the other facilities needed, to rehabilitate people with head injuries.

6. Job opportunities. A person who has had a head injury often cannot be found work. The cause is partly that the victim may have less tolerance of fatigue and stress, and often has behavioural problems. Much of the difficulty is due to prejudice on the part of employers.
Action: Employers must be educated to recognize that a person who has had a head injury has a worthwhile potential, provided that allowance is made for him. The employer should be given incentives to provide the conditions in which the victim can be employed to the profit of the employer and the advantage of the employee.

7. Occupation for a person for whom a job cannot be found. Some people who have had head injuries will not be able to work in a commercial environment, because of physical, intellectual, or behavioural problems. The victim in this position needs an occupation as a source of satisfaction, to give structure to his days, and to provide him with social relationships.
Action: From a drop-in centre to sheltered workshops, a range of opportunities is needed for head-injured people who cannot work in a normal environment. Some of these are best supplied by the voluntary agencies such as head-injury societies, others such as sheltered workshops require institutional or government support.

> **Management needs—third stage**
> Vocational rehabilitation
> Job opportunity
> A place with dignity for those who cannot work

8. Major behavioural problems. A few people who have had head injuries are left with major problems of behaviour which need full-time professional care for treatment with the hope of return to normal life, or occasionally for long terms. This is a psychiatric problem, but in many places psychiatric services are unable to provide for the victim.

Action: Psychiatric services are needed for people with serious behavioural problems following head injury, to allow them to live in safety and with reasonable dignity and comfort.

9. Persisting problems after mild head injuries. It is becoming recognized that 5–10 per cent of people who suffer mild head injury have difficulties in getting back to normal function and employment and that their problems may last from a few weeks to several years. The psychological and medical services in many places are not able to deal with the problems.

Action: Mild head-injury clinics are needed, attached to the accident services of all but the smallest hospital centres.

> **Management needs—areas often neglected**
> Mild head injury
> Severe behavioural problems
> Do not let the head-injured victim be written off

PRESENTING NEEDS TO THE AUTHORITIES

In many places the needs of head-injured victims are not being met. Some parts of the service as we have outlined it above may not be available, and often there is no central organization to make sure that everyone works together. Anyone who attends a meeting of head-injured people and their families will recognize that there is a majority of dissatisfied customers.

The authorities that run accident and rehabilitation services vary from place to place, but the arguments which affect them are likely to be the same everywhere. The authorities will take some humane notice of the amount of suffering experienced but they will need other reasons to give priority to any area. Usually they will be most influenced by the cost of any extensions of their existing service and they will not agree to increased funding unless it can be shown that obvious gains can be set against this. In preparing an argument, the first need then is to know the numbers and severity of the injuries in your community, with an estimate of the human cost; deaths, family disruptions, days off work, and any other information you can supply.

The authority will need a reason for priority. It may say that it cannot single out one service for improvement. You can then argue that head injury is a consequence of the modern way of living and therefore that the community has a special responsibility. You can point out that there is no doubt that the community inherits special problems when head injuries are poorly rehabilitated, in the shape of long-term disability and the need to make provision for people whose thinking and behaviour remain disturbed.

Economic arguments will be powerful. It will be useful to have an estimate of the current cost of handling head injuries, and to make a reasonable prediction of the savings that might be made by improving the service. The inefficiency of using acute hospital beds for long-term care, and the saving from provision of less-expensive rehabilitation beds is a good argument in some places. It is more difficult to give exact figures for the saving in the period of disability which can result from good rehabilitation, but the general argument can be put forcefully. This may be more telling when dealing with insurers, who bear the burden of long disability, rather than the hospital authorities.

The figures presented here may be useful as a starting point. We collected the information from a survey in Auckland, New Zealand, a city of 850 000 people; the figures seem to be comparable, for example, with figures reported from San Diego and the UK.

> **Figures for numbers of head injuries and hospital use from a Survey in Auckland, New Zealand, in 1986.**
>
> These are expressed as numbers per 100 000 of population per year.
>
> Admitted to hospital:
> with a primary diagnosis of head injury;   65
> with severe multiple injuries and head injury;   5.4
> with other injuries but also a head injury;   57
>
> Seen at hospital but not admitted: 654
>
> Hospital bed-days occupied—primary head injury
> and severe multiple injuries: 4,700
>
> With persisting problems after mild head injury
> (⅔ with problems continuing more than 1 month):   30

Lastly, the professionals who are involved should be mobilized to help. This together with strong public pressure is able to produce results. The Royal College of Physicians of London commissioned a report on physical disability in young people which has been very influential. In 1986 it made strong recommendations on the need for services for head-injured victims, particularly for a central organizing body in each area. Many other professional bodies in the UK, the USA, Australia, and elsewhere have made similar recommendations. The way public support can be organized and who can be persuaded to lend themselves to a movement of this sort will be different in every area. The originators will usually be the families and victims who have come together to form head-injury societies, and they will have to mobilize every source of help they can. Good luck to them!

> **Organizing a head-injury service requires commitment from:**
> the head injured
> their families
> concerned professionals
> the public
> politicians

12. Suggestions for further reading

FOR THE NON-SPECIALIST, NON-MEDICAL READER

Weiss, L., Thatch, D., and Thatch, J., with Gray, L. (1983). *I wasn't finished with life*. E. Hart Press, Dallas, Texas.

Sitkin, L.A. and Murdoch, B.E. (1987). *Brain injury and the family*. Simmons and Hall, San Francisco.

FOR THE NON-SPECIALIST MEDICAL OR PARAMEDICAL READER

Levin, H.S., Eisenberg, H.M., and Benton, A.L. (ed). (1989). *Mild Head Injury*. Oxford University Press, New York.

Lezak, M. (ed). (1989). *Assessment of the behavioural consequences of head-injury*. Alan R. Liss, New York.

FOR THE SPECIALIST MEDICAL OR PARAMEDICAL READER

Brooks, N. (ed). (1984). *Closed head injury: psychological, social, and family consequences*. Oxford University Press, New York.

Levin, H.S., Grafman, J., and Eisenberg, H.M. (ed). (1987). *Neurobehavioural recovery from head injury*. Oxford University Press, New York.

Royal College of Physicians Committee on the Young Physically Disabled. (1986). *Report. Journal of the Royal College of Physicians of London*, **20** 160-94.

Appendix A: Glossary

Ageusia. Partial or total loss of the sense of taste.

Agnosia. Partial or total loss of the ability to know the meaning or significance of things. It can affect experience of things seen, heard, touched, smelt, or tasted.

Agraphia. Partial or total loss of the ability to express oneself in writing.

Alexia. Partial or total loss of reading skills. It can affect understanding of written language, symbols, or music scores.

Amnesia. Partial or total loss of the ability to recall things which have been done or experienced. (See also retrograde or pre-traumatic amnesia, and post-traumatic amnesia.)

Anarthria. Loss of speech through impairment of muscle control, caused by injury to the nerves supplying the speech muscles.

Anosmia. Partial or total loss of the sense of smell.

Anticonvulsants. Medication prescribed to control epileptic seizures.

Aphasia. Partial or complete impairment of the ability to make oneself understood, or to understand others through language, caused by injury to the brain. It can affect speaking, writing, sign language, reading, or listening.

Anoxia. Lack of oxygen supply to brain cells.

Apraxia. Partial or total loss of the ability to perform purposeful movements while still having the ability to move and to be aware of the movement.

Ataxia. Lack of movement co-ordination, due to brain injury.

Brain stem. Part of the brain which connects the cerebral hemispheres with the spinal cord. It contains control centres for vital organs such as the heart and the lungs.

Burr hole. A hole drilled in the skull.

Central nervous system (CNS). The brain and spinal cord.

Cerebellum. Part of the brain sited at the base of the brain behind the brain stem. It is important for the control of movement.

CAT Scan. Computerized axial tomography, a special X-ray procedure which gives a picture of soft tissues as well as bone.

Cerebral cortex. The folded ridged grey matter on the surface of the cerebral hemispheres.

Cerebral hemispheres. The two side-by-side halves of the cerebrum, the main part of the brain.

Cerebro-spinal fluid (CSF). The clear colourless fluid in the spaces inside and around the brain and spinal cord.

Cerebrum. The main part of the brain which sits in the upper part of the skull cavity.

Closed head injury. Damage to the brain which is not accompanied by a penetrating injury.

Coma. An altered state of consciousness where the person cannot be aroused.

Concussion. Altered consciousness caused by jarring of the brain; for example, from a blow or a fall.

Contusion. Bruising of the brain matter.

Cranium. The bony skull.

Debridement. Surgical removal of dead tissue and foreign matter from a wound.

Diplopia. Double vision.

Dura mater. The outermost of the three membranes covering the brain.

Dysarthria. Impairment of speech caused by faulty speech muscle movements.

Dysgraphia. See Agraphia.

Dysphasia. See Aphasia.

Dyspraxia. See Apraxia.

Edema. See Oedema.

Electroencephalogram (EEG). A procedure where the changes in the electrical potentials in the brain are recorded.

Evoked potentials. Responses to signals (either sounds, or lights, or touch) which are recorded from the brain by special EEG techniques.

Extradural. Between the dura and the skull.

Frontal lobe. The part of each cerebral hemisphere primarily concerned with the control and regulation of behaviour.

Haematoma. A collection or clot of blood.

Haemorrhage. Bleeding.

Hematoma. See haematoma.

Hemianopia. Loss of sight in one half of the visual field.

Hemineglect. Loss of attention for things in one half of space.

Hemiparesis. Weakness of one side of the body.

Hemiplegia. Paralysis of one side of the body.

Hemorrhage. See Haemorrhage.

Hydrocephalus. An accumulation of cerebrospinal fluid within the ventricles of the brain.

Infarct. An area where brain cells have died as a result of loss of blood supply.

Intracranial pressure (ICP). The pressure inside the head.

Nasogastric tube. A tube inserted into the stomach through the nose to allow nourishment.

Neuron. A nerve cell.

Occipital lobe. The part of each cerebral hemisphere primarily concerned with perception and interpretation of visual information.

Oedema. Excessive accumulation of fluid in the tissue as a result of traumatic injury.

Parietal lobe. The part of each cerebral hemisphere primarily concerned with the perception and interpretation of sensations and movement.

Photophobia. Abnormal sensitivity of the eyes to light.

Post-traumatic amnesia (PTA). Inability to remember events that happen after a blow to the head which causes an alteration of consciousness, even when the victim is apparently awake.

Pre-traumatic amnesia. See Retrograde amnesia.

Retrograde amnesia. Inability to remember events that happened for a period before a blow to the head that caused an alteration of consciousness.

Subdural. Between the dura and the brain.

Temporal lobe. The part of each cerebral hemisphere concerned with sound interpretation and perception, and important in memory function.

Tracheotomy. An operation to make a opening in the windpipe to allow breathing.

Ventricle. Fluid-filled cavity in the brain.

Appendix B: Contacts for family support groups

Contact persons and addresses of local support groups are liable to change frequently and so the address and phone number of the parent association has been given. The parent organization will be able to provide information about what is available in different areas in the country and an up-to-date contact.

GREAT BRITAIN

The National Head Injuries Association (Headway), 17–21 Clumber Avenue, Sherwood Rise, Nottingham NG5 1AG, UK. Phone: (0602) 622382

UNITED STATES OF AMERICA

National Head Injury Foundation (Inc), 333 Turnpike Road, Southborough, MA 01772, USA. Phone: (508) 485-9950 Family Help Line: 1-800-444-NHIF

AUSTRALIA

The Head Injury Council of Australia (HICOA), PO Box 304, Port Melbourne 3207, Australia. Phone: (03) 696-1388

This body represents all state head injury organizations, and supplied the following addresses of associated state groups.

Kel Buchanan, Vice President HICOA, Administrator, Head Injury Society of Western Australia, PO Box 298, Applecross 6154, Australia. Phone: (09) 3306370

Alana Clohesy, Director, Headway New South Wales, PO Box 424, Burwood 2134, Australia. Phone: (02) 7472866

Alwyn Ricci, President, Headway Queensland, 38 Flower Street, Nundah 4012, Australia. Phone: (07) 2667664

Frank Quigley, President, Head Injury Society of South Australia, PO Box 20, Stepney 5069, Australia. Phone: (08) 2646275

NEW ZEALAND

Sara-Jane Fleming, Secretary, Head Injury Society of New Zealand, 2/194 Barnard Street, Wadestown, Wellington, New Zealand. Phone: (04) 499-0551

Index